Andrei Zbuchea

Osteoarticular injuries due to electrical aggression

AF141895

Andrei Zbuchea

Osteoarticular injuries due to electrical aggression

LAP LAMBERT Academic Publishing

Impressum / Imprint

Bibliografische Information der Deutschen Nationalbibliothek: Die Deutsche Nationalbibliothek verzeichnet diese Publikation in der Deutschen Nationalbibliografie; detaillierte bibliografische Daten sind im Internet über http://dnb.d-nb.de abrufbar.

Alle in diesem Buch genannten Marken und Produktnamen unterliegen warenzeichen-, marken- oder patentrechtlichem Schutz bzw. sind Warenzeichen oder eingetragene Warenzeichen der jeweiligen Inhaber. Die Wiedergabe von Marken, Produktnamen, Gebrauchsnamen, Handelsnamen, Warenbezeichnungen u.s.w. in diesem Werk berechtigt auch ohne besondere Kennzeichnung nicht zu der Annahme, dass solche Namen im Sinne der Warenzeichen- und Markenschutzgesetzgebung als frei zu betrachten wären und daher von jedermann benutzt werden dürften.

Bibliographic information published by the Deutsche Nationalbibliothek: The Deutsche Nationalbibliothek lists this publication in the Deutsche Nationalbibliografie; detailed bibliographic data are available in the Internet at http://dnb.d-nb.de.

Any brand names and product names mentioned in this book are subject to trademark, brand or patent protection and are trademarks or registered trademarks of their respective holders. The use of brand names, product names, common names, trade names, product descriptions etc. even without a particular marking in this work is in no way to be construed to mean that such names may be regarded as unrestricted in respect of trademark and brand protection legislation and could thus be used by anyone.

Coverbild / Cover image: www.ingimage.com

Verlag / Publisher:
LAP LAMBERT Academic Publishing
ist ein Imprint der / is a trademark of
OmniScriptum GmbH & Co. KG
Bahnhofstraße 28, 66111 Saarbrücken, Deutschland / Germany
Email: info@lap-publishing.com

Herstellung: siehe letzte Seite /
Printed at: see last page
ISBN: 978-3-659-83533-9

Copyright © 2016 OmniScriptum GmbH & Co. KG
Alle Rechte vorbehalten. / All rights reserved. Saarbrücken 2016

Osteoarticular Injuries Due to Electrical Aggression

Andrei Zbuchea, MD, PhD
Chief of Plastic Surgery Department
County Emergency Hospital
Ploiesti, Romania

1

Table of Contents

Introduction

The electricity represents an intimate and indispensable part of our own culture, civilization and technology. Nevertheless, the electrical aggression is one of the most serious and devastating challenge over the human organism. The electrical flow can determine not only apparent deep burns of the contact areas, but especially profound and progressive deteriorations of the internal tissues and organs, which are disguised by the external lesions, which worsen the prognosis and which require dynamic, prompt and complex treatment.

Regarding the external insults, WHO defines burn as "an injury to the skin or other organic tissue primarily caused by heat or due to radiation, radioactivity, electricity, friction or contact with chemicals" (1, 2).

Globally, burns represent a serious public health problem, with an estimated 265,000 deaths each year, the majority occurring in low- and middle-income countries. Non-fatal burns are also an important cause of morbidity and disability, with significant economic, social and psychological impact. In 2004, nearly 11 million people all over the world require medical attention due to burn lesions. In India, over one million people suffer moderately or severely burns every year (1).

According to data provided by ABA, in 2015 in USA were nearly half a million burn injuries receiving medical treatment, and 40,000 hospitalizations related to burn injury, including 30,000 at hospital burn centers, with a survival rate 96.7%. The admission causes in American hospitals were mainly fire/flame (43%) and scald (34%), and only 4% electrical (3).

The electrical burns were classified in two main categories, as follows:
- burns caused by electrical arc (flash/flame), without an electrical current flow through the human body
- burns through electrocution, with entrance and exit sites

After according first aid, the electrical burns, including lighting injury, should always be referred to a burn centre or to a specialized burn care service, for improving the prognosis and the final outcome (4-6).

The electrical injuries can be classified according to a series of parameters (7):
- The power source: electrical or lightning
- The voltage: low or high voltage
- The type of current: alternating or direct.

Each type of electrical injury has a specific injury pattern, prognosis and therapeutic management. The spectrum of electrical injuries is very broad, spreading from minimal injury, to extensive burns, severe multiorgan insults and even death. Approximately 20% of all electrical injuries occur in children, which are mostly injured at home, with extension cords (60-70%) and wall outlets (10-15%) being clearly the most common sources. Furthermore, the electrical burns constitute 2-3% of all burns in children that require emergency room care. In adults, most electrical injuries occur at the workplace and represent the fourth leading cause of job-related traumatic death. Approximately one third of all electrical traumas and most high-voltage injuries are work related. Majority of these occupational electrocutions result from power line contact (5-6% of all work-related deaths), whereas 25% are due to utilization of electrical tools or machines. The annual occupational death rate from electricity is 1 death per 100,000 workers, with a male-to-female ratio of 9:1 (7-9).

In USA, the electrical injuries have a mortality rate of 3-5%, but up to 40% of serious cases are fatal; they result in about 1000 deaths per year and 3000 admissions to specialized burn centers per year. Moreover, in USA, lightning injury causes 50-300 deaths per year, encountered more on people being wet or carrying a metal object (7-9).

Broadly, the electrical injuries can be divided in four classes, as follows:
- Electrocutions (true electrical injuries), when the electric flow passes through the human body, entrance and exit sites being encountered
- Flash injuries, when no electrical energy goes through the skin and appear partial thickness burns, due to electrical arc
- Flame injuries, due to ignition of the clothing by electrical arc; electricity may or may not traverse the human body
- Lighting injuries, a particular type of electric flow which appears at extremely high voltages for the shortest duration (9).

Electrical injuries have a wide range of acute and chronic manifestations, not seen with other types of thermal injury. Morbidity, length of hospital stay, complications, resources involved and amplitude of therapeutic procedures are much higher than those expected, based only on cutaneous burn size (10).

The electrical injuries are not very common trauma, but the emergency departments are constantly confronted with such injuries, with a specific pathophysiology and with high morbidity and mortality. Clinical manifestations vary considerably, from transient unpleasant sensations without apparent injury, to extensive tissue damage (9).

Although electrical burns represent only 3- 4% of all burn injuries, they consume enormous amounts of material and human resources and also require a carefully planned team approach for optimal care (10). Electrical injuries can determine large tissue loss, often leading to amputation of involved extremities, besides other harmful complications: renal, septic, cardiovascular, neurological, osteoarticular and ocular manifestations (10, 11). Thorough knowledge of the pathophysiology and of the optimal treatment guidelines improves patient care, final outcome and quality of life (9).

Chapter 1 Pathophysiology of electrical lesions

The clinical action of electricity is determined by the directional flow of electrons across a potential gradient from high to low concentration, through a conductive material (human tissues and organs). The voltage (V) represents the magnitude of this potential difference and is usually generated by the electrical source (7).

The type, extent and severity of the electrical lesions are determined by a series of **parameters**, including (7-10):
- Voltage
- Current strength (amperage)
- Type of current (alternating or direct)
- Pathway of current flow
- Duration of contact with the source
- Tissues resistance at the areas of contact and passage
- Individual susceptibility.

Voltage (V)

According to voltage, the electrical lesions are usually divided as low-voltage and high-voltage injuries, using a threshold of 500 V or 1000 V (7, 9, 10, 12). High morbidity and mortality has been reported in 600V direct current injury, associated with railroad "third rail" contact (7).

In general, the high voltage current is responsible for greater morbidity and mortality than the low-voltage current, although some fatal injury can appear at household current (110 to 240 V) (9). The most serious and mutilating types of electrical injuries results from high-voltage electrical currents (typically more than 500 volts) passing through the human body. Since the current passes deep to the skin, the magnitude, extent and severity of the electrical lesions are often underestimated. These high-voltage injuries determine major tissue destruction, possibly leading to limb amputations, and require special expertise and prompt treatment (12).

Low-voltage injuries are also denominated as low-tension injuries; this category comprises most injuries caused by household current, such as (13):
- the child who bites into the cord producing lip, face and tongue injuries
- occupational injuries resulting from the use of small power tools
- those who become grounded while touching an object that is energized.

Nearly all burn lesions occurring indoors, with the exception of those due to specialized industrial settings, belong to the low-voltage type (10).

Low voltage burns are mostly generated in the area immediately surrounding the contact injury. Instead, at high voltage injuries, the apparent cutaneous burns are often associated with deep, extensive, underlying tissue damage, very closely resembling a crush injury (10).

High-voltage injuries are also denominated as high-tension injuries. Most frequently, they are the result of occupational exposure to outside power lines and in a great measure they occur when the patient touches an overhead high voltage power line, through a conductive object. Rarely, patients get into electrical switching equipment and directly touch energized component (13).

Lightning injuries are usually classified separately and they involve voltages much higher than those of the two previous injuries. The typical lightning injury involves energy with high voltage and high amperage, but extremely short duration. Lightning is a unidirectional massive flow of current that runs from 1/10 to 1/1000 of a second, but often has voltages which can exceed even 10 million volts. The most significant difference between lightning and high-voltage electrical injuries is done by the duration of exposure to the current. Generally, the lightning represents a unidirectional massive current impulse and is best understood as a current rather than a voltage phenomenon. The largest flow of electrical current drains into the ground, before much of it passes through and along the human body. Lightning injuries occur mostly when the patient is part of or near the lightning bolt, and generally, the patient was the tallest object around or near a tall object, such as a tree (9, 13).

Other electrical injuries are represented by intentional injuries, due to (13):
- the use of high-voltage devices for rapid incapacitation, child and/or spouse abuse, and torture
- the use of skin electrodes in medicine, that can cause a perimeter effect.

Current strength (amperage, A)

The current intensity (I) represents the volume of electrons flowing across the potential gradient and is measured in amperes (A). It is a measure of the amount of energy that flows through a human body. Energy is perceptible to the touch at a current as low as a threshold of 1 mA. A narrow range exists between perceptible current and the "let go" current, which is the maximum current at which a person can grasp and then release the current before muscle tetany develops and makes it impossible to let go (7).

All tissue lesions and systemic effects are directly proportional to the magnitude of current delivered to the victim. According to Ohm's law, current flow (amperage) is directly proportional to voltage and inversely proportional to tissue resistance (9):

Ohm's law: I=V/R
where: I=current, V=voltage, R=resistance.

Of the all three parameters encountered in Ohm's law, usually only voltage can be determined in current practice and is used to estimate the potential magnitude of current exposure and, therefore, the magnitude of injury (9). While the patient or witnesses often knows the voltage implicated, the intensity of current remains practically unknown (10).

Also, there may be individual variation on the energy dose required for a specific effect. For instance, less energy is generally more harmful in children, who have more water content and thinner skin and, consequently, better conductivity and less resistance, and in patients under moist conditions (9).

The values of current intensity required for some specific and expected clinical manifestations are delineated in Table 1, for 60 Hz current (7, 9, 13):

Table 1: Effects of different current intensities

Current intensity	Event
1 mA	Threshold of perception, probable tingling sensation
3-5 mA	"Let go" current for an average child
6-8 mA	"Let go" current for an average woman
7-9 mA	"Let go" current for an average man
16 mA	Maximum current a person can grasp and "let go"
16-20 mA	Tetany of skeletal muscles
20-50 mA	Paralysis of respiratory muscles (respiratory arrest)
50-100 mA	Threshold for ventricular fibrillation
> 2 A	Asystole
6 A	Defibrillation
15-30 A	Common household circuit breakers

Type of current (alternating or direct)

Electrical current is further classified as direct current (DC) or alternating current (AC). The direct current flows in the same direction unceasingly, as the current which is generated by batteries. In the alternating current, the flow of electrons changes direction rhythmically, with constant and specific frequency, such as household electricity largely available. Thus, AC is the most common type of electricity provided in homes and offices, with a standardized frequency of 50 or 60 cycles/sec (Hz) (7, 13).

AC, which is used widely, is by far more dangerous than DC. High voltage DC tends to cause a single violent muscle contraction, often strong enough to throw the victim away from the electrical source, thus resulting in brief duration of contact with the source. In contrast, AC of the same voltage is considered to be approximately 3 times more dangerous than DC, because the cyclic flow of electrons can cause continuing, tetanic muscle contraction, often preventing the patient from releasing his grip on the electrical source and, thereby, increasing the duration of contact and current delivery. Muscle tetany occurs when fibers are stimulated at a frequency ranging from 40 to 110 Hz; the standard frequency of 50 or 60 Hz of household current is within that register. If the patient's hand get in touch with the electrical source, when tetanic muscle contraction occur, then the extremity flexors contract, causing the victim to grasp the current and resulting in prolonged contact with the source.

In consequence, the electrical exposure may be prolonged and therefore, the harmful effects will be amplified. Even a small intensity of alternating current, merely enough to be felt as a mild shock, can cause a definitely patient's grip. Slightly more alternating current can cause respiratory arrest, due to thoracic muscle tetany involving the diaphragm and intercostal muscles, making breathing impossible. Still more intense current can cause fatal heart rhythms. The repetitive nature of AC increases the likelihood of current delivery to the myocardium during the vulnerable recovery period of the cardiac cycle, which can precipitate ventricular fibrillation (7, 9, 13).

Pathway of current flow

The electrical current pathway determines which tissues and organs are vulnerable and what type of injury can be encountered. The most common entry point for electrical current is the hand, and the second most common is the head. On the other side, the most common exit point is the foot. A current that passes from an arm to another or from an arm to a leg may travel through the heart and is much more dangerous than a current that goes between a leg and the ground. Thus, electrical current that passes through the head or thorax are more likely to produce some fatal injury.

Transthoracic currents are expected to cause:
- fatal arrhythmia
- direct cardiac damage
- respiratory arrest.
On the other hand, a current that travels through the head can cause:
- direct brain injury
- seizure
- respiratory arrest
- paralysis.

Electrothermal tissue injury results in tissue edema and necrosis; therefore, the development of a compartment syndrome can occur in any compartment of the human body. Nevertheless, the extremities and especially the legs are the locations most commonly encountered for the appearance and progression of a compartment syndrome, which represents an emergency which require early diagnosis and prompt, dynamic and appropriate treatment (9, 13).

Duration of contact with the source

Obviously, the severity of electrical lesions is directly proportional with the duration of contact with the source, as well as the passage time through the different parts of the human body. Prolonged tetanic muscle contractions are more deleterious than a unique violent muscle contraction, resulting in the disengagement of the electrical power source. The most significant difference between lightning and high-voltage electrical injuries is done by the duration of exposure to the electrical current (9). Also, in about one half of high voltage victims, altered levels of consciousness can contribute to prolonged periods of electrical contact (10).

Tissues resistance at the areas of contact and passage

The resistance (R) is the impedance to flow of electrons across a gradient and it varies depending on the electrolyte and water content of the human body tissue at the contact areas or through which electrical current is passing (7).

The resistance of the human body varies considerably between different tissues and organs. In general, tissues with high fluid and electrolyte content conduct electricity better. Bones are the most resistant tissues to the flow of electricity. Nerve tissue is the least resistant, and together with blood vessels, muscles, and mucous membranes, due to high electrolyte and water content, they provide low resistance and they are excellent conductors of electricity. Skin provides intermediate resistance and represents the most important factor hindering current flow. Skin at the areas of contact provides the primary resistor against electrical current, and its degree of resistance is determined by its thickness and moisture. Hardly thick or calloused areas of skin are excellent resistors; whereas a moderate amount of water or sweat on the skin surface can lower its resistance significantly. Thus, skin resistance varies from 1000 ohms for low resistance humid thin skin to several thousand ohms for dry calloused skin (7, 9). Skin resistance at the point of contact ranges from very low values for sweat-soaked hands or skin in the summer to more than 100 000 ohms for heavily calloused hands or feet during very dry winter weather. Individual susceptibility is a non-quantifiable parameter used to explain why two or more patients, exposed to the same condition, have extremely different injuries (10).

The pathophysiological significance of the tissue resistance resides in the generation and spreading of more heat in a more resistant conductor (tissue) than in a less resistant conductor, following the passage of a given current. As stated above, resistance is the ability to impede the flow of electricity. The direct dissipation of energy as heat is designated joule heating, and represents the major cause of thermal burns to skin and profound tissues. This engendered heat is directly proportional to the resistance of the tissue through which the current is travelling and to the duration of contact as dictated by Joule's law:

Joule's law: $E = IVT = I^2RT$
where E=energy, I= current, R= resistance and T= duration of contact.

Therefore, tissues that are less conductive and more resistant are likely to heat up more, as electrical current passes through them. The order of tissues, ranging from the most conductive (i.e., least resistant) to the least conductive (i.e., most resistant) is illustrated in Table 2 (13).

Table 2: The range of tissues, from the most conductive (least resistant) to the least conductive (most resistant).

Resistance	Tissue
Least	Nerves
	Blood
	Mucous membranes
	Muscle
Intermediate	Dry skin
	Tendon
	Fat
Most	Bone

Most of the human body's resistance is concentrated in the skin. Therefore, the thicker and dryer the skin, the greater will be its resistance. The skin's resistance decreases greatly when it became broken or wet. If skin resistance is high, more of the damage due to electrical injury is local, producing only skin burns. On the other hand, if skin resistance is low, wet or broken skin, more of the damage affects the profound organs (13).

Also, the experimental studies performed on laboratory animals have demonstrated that resistance varies continuously with time, initially dropping slowly, then much more abruptly, until arcing occurs at the contact sites. Resistance then rises to infinity and current flow ceases. The measurements of the body temperature, taken simultaneously, showed that rate of temperature rise parallels changes in amperage. The tissue temperature was the critical factor in the magnitude and severity of tissue damage. Interestingly, there wasn't put into evidence any increase in temperature distal to the contact points (10).

The degree and the severity of electrical lesions are together predicted and established by **all previously expounded parameters**, such as: magnitude of energy delivered, resistance encountered, conductance, current pathway, and duration of contact. Systemic effects and tissue damage are directly proportional to the magnitude of current delivered to the victim. According to Ohm's law, current intensity is directly related to voltage and inversed to resistance (13).

The three major mechanisms of electrical injuries are as follows:
1. Direct cellular and tissue damage, by:
- the impairment of the physiologic conduction systems, such as cardiac contraction and diaphragm excursion, which can lead to arrhythmia and apnea
- the electroporation or the electropermeabilization of the cell membranes, which can lead to the deterioration of transmembranar exchanges, intracellular ion and protein balance, and finally apoptosis
- altering cell membrane resting potential
- eliciting tetany.
2. Conversion of electrical energy into thermal energy, through joule heating, which can lead to extensive tissue destruction and coagulation necrosis.
3. Mechanical injury with direct trauma due to a fall or to violent muscle contraction and implicated in osteo-articular lesions (9, 13, 14).

The local electric field can provide sufficient magnitude to determine electrical breakdown of cell membranes and subsequent cell lysis. In theory, large cells such as muscle and nerve cells are more vulnerable to electrical damage. The clinical evidence that further suggests the breakdown and rupture of muscle and nerve cell membranes by electrical trauma is:
- The release of myoglobin in large amounts, from within the intracellular space;
- The intense spasm and rigor commonly described by people involved, which suggest that the muscle cell is depolarized and maybe that cytoplasmic ATP levels are inadequate to dissociate the actinmyosin complex;
- The elevated plasma levels of arachidonic acid derivatives of membrane phospholipids;
- The delayed paralysis and nerve cell death, even years after electrical trauma in which the thermal injury component was practically absent;
- The particular vulnerability of large cells to injury (13).

When an electrical current is transferred to the human body through direct contact with a conducting material or an arc that reaches the skin surface, the electrons begin to flow, as ions flow in a solution. Flow can be divided into:

13

1. direct type
2. indirect type
3. an arc.

1. Direct flow is the most common type and it happens when the patient touches a conductor, causing contact burns.

2. Indirect flow occurs in flashovers, in which the flow of current proceeds along the external surface of the body and is enhanced by wet skin or clothing. Flash (also called side flash, flash discharge, splash, or spray) occurs when current begins down one path, such as a tree, then jumps to a grounded nearby person, following the path of least resistance. This mechanism is believed to be the most encountered in lightning strike injuries.

3. An arc is one of the types of electrical flow that provokes the greatest amounts of current and heat; it is a current spark formed between two objects of differing potential that are not in contact with each other, usually a highly charged source and a ground. An arc results when a stream of plasma (a highly ionized gaseous- good conductor) is generated from the atoms in the conducting material. The formation of an arc depends on the voltage and the dielectric properties of the insulating medium, usually air. In patients with a high-voltage injury, an arc is usually produced before they make physical contact with the electrical source, and they are in the circuit. The temperature of an arc can reach up to $2500\text{-}10000^\circ C$ (13).

From pathophysiological point of view, the electrical injuries can involve multiple mechanisms and body systems. Entry and exit areas fail to reflect the real magnitude of underlying tissue damage, as electrical current can cause multiple and extensive injuries, at distance from its apparent pathway through the patient. Electrical flows are capable of damaging cells and tissues through both thermal and nonthermal mechanisms. While joule heating is a certain and clear mechanism, which is generally recognized as the main factor to mediate tissue injury in electrical trauma, the possible roles of electrical breakdown of cell membranes and cell lysis have not yet been thoroughly considered and explained. The literature on the pathophysiology of electrical injuries has been inconclusive; there have been proposed a series of interpretations and theories. In fact, the exact pathophysiology of electrical injury is not well understood due to the large number of variables that cannot be measured or controlled, when an electrical current passes through human tissues (13).

Chapter 2 Clinical manifestations of electrical lesions

The electrical lesions may have a very wide variety of clinical forms and presentations, depending on the parameters discussed in the previous chapter, such as voltage, current, pathway, duration of contact, and type of circuit.

Besides these, different tissues and organs exhibit specific susceptibility, resistance and pattern of injury to electrical damage, as follows in Table 3 (13).

Table 3: Tissue damage according to the level of injury

Pattern of injury	Tissue damage
Skin	flash burns, thermal burns, arc burns, linear burns, contact electrical burns
Muscle	swell, pain, contractions, spasms, myonecrosis, compartment syndrome
Blood vessels	blood cloths, microvascular deterioration, myoglobinemia, vasoconstriction, thrombosis, ischemia
Heart	arrhythmia, asystolia, cardiac arrest, ventricular fibrillation, sinus tachycardia, myocardial necrosis/infarction
Nerves	weakness, paralysis, tingling, numbness, uncontrollable loss of urine (incontinence), and chronic pain
Brain	seizures, hemorrhages, poor short-term memory, unconsciousness, ischemia, personality changes, difficulty sleeping, irritability
Bones	joint dislocations, fractures, other blunt injuries
Kidney	myoglobinuria, acute renal failure, acute tubular necrosis
Ears	perforation of the eardrum, hemorrhagia
Eyes	cataracts

Clinical presentations range from a tingling sensation, to a widespread tissue damage and even to sudden death (15). Electrical injuries can present with a large variety of aspects, including cardiac or respiratory arrest, coma, blunt trauma, and severe burns of several types (7).

For the proper and adequate management of the electrical lesions, there is extremely important to truly establish from the beginning:
- type of electrical exposure (AC or DC; high or low voltage)
- pathway through the human body
- duration of contact
- concurrent trauma.

Low-voltage AC injury without loss of consciousness and/or arrest
These injuries are exposures of less than 1000V and usually appear in the home or office setting. Currently, children with electrical injuries present after biting or chewing on an electrical cord and suffer oral burns. These types of electrical injuries can be also encountered in adults working on home appliances or electrical circuits. Low-voltage AC can lead to significant injury in case of prolonged, tetanic muscle contraction.

Low-voltage AC injury with loss of consciousness and/or arrest
An electrical exposure may be difficult to diagnose in respiratory arrest or ventricular fibrillation that is not witnessed. All unwitnessed and unconfirmed arrests should include this possibility in the differential diagnosis. Emergency personnel, family and co-workers should be queried about this possibility. If a scream was heard before the patient's collapse, this may be due to involuntary contraction of chest wall muscles from electrical current.

High-voltage AC injury without loss of consciousness and/or arrest
Typically, high-voltage injuries do not determine loss of consciousness or arrest, but instead cause devastating thermal burns. In occupational exposures, magnitude of voltage can be obtained from the local power supply company.

High-voltage AC injury with loss of consciousness and/or arrest
This is an occasional manifestation of high-voltage AC injuries, which do not frequently lead to loss of consciousness. Accurate history is necessary to be obtained from bystanders or from emergency personnel.

Direct current (DC) injury
These injuries typically lead to a single and strong muscle contraction, which throws the victim away from the electrical source. They are exceptionally associated with loss of consciousness unless there is severe head trauma, and victims can usually provide their own history (7).

Altogether, low-voltage currents tend to cause less global morbidity than high-voltage, but it is extremely important to establish by accurate history that a apparently low-voltage burn was not in reality caused by a high-voltage source (like a microwave, computer, TV monitor, or any other device that enhances voltage through a transformer). Furthermore, low-voltage burns can still cause cardiac arrhythmias, seizures, and long-term complications, especially if contact is established near the chest or head (7).

The external resistance to electric flow is provided primarily by the skin and appendages and forwards by the internal resistance of all other internal tissues, including nerves, blood, muscles, tendons, fat and bone. Whereas the skin resistance can be altered by moisture, a great deal of electric flow can be transmitted to deeper tissues and organs, before significant skin damage will be ascertained. Thus, electric current may be retained in the bones, transforming into heat and leading to necrosis and coagulation of small- to medium-sized vessels within the muscles and other tissues, almost entirely avoiding the skin.

Mostly, the main symptom of an electrical injury is a skin burn. A specific type of burn, so-called the "kissing burn," occurs at the flexor creases of limbs and is due to the current passing through the opposing skin at the joint when the flexor muscles contract due to tetany. Not all electrical exposures cause external lesions; high-voltage exposures may lead to edema, extensive and widespread internal burns, coagulation necrosis and compartment syndrome. Lightning injury typically determines superficial surface burns (9).

Depending on the previously discussed parameters, electrical exposures can lead to a variety of burns and other traumatic injuries, as well as multiorgan dysfunction. A thorough and complete physical examination is strictly required, in order to assess the full extent of electrical injuries. Occupational injuries have a great presumption of future litigation, and physical examination findings should be documented with photographs if possible, with the proper releases, and should be recorded in the patient's medical documents (7).

In the following, the most frequently and representative lesions caused by electrical exposures will be highlighted, ranked by the pattern of injury.

Skin – different types of electrical burns

According to voltage, current strength, pathway, duration of contact, and type of circuit, electrical exposures can cause a variety of burns, through several different mechanisms. Thermal injuries due to electrical aggression are often the most severe and disabling consequences of electricity, after cardiac arrhythmias, and their aspect may initially appear minor and trivial, despite significant deep tissue injury subsequently requiring fasciotomy, aggressive debridements or amputation. Burns are often most severe at the source and ground contact areas; the source is usually the hands or the head while the ground is often in the feet. The current strength and duration of contact with the electrical source greatly determine the severity and extent of tissue damage, as well as the prognosis. All electrical burns should be carefully documented and, if possible, photographed, taking into account the possible unfavourable evolution and the medico-legal concerns (7).

High-voltage burns

Typically, these lesions show a contact point where the patient touched the circuit and a ground point. High-voltage burns can cause significant damage to underlying profound tissues, while significantly sparing the outer surface of the skin. These burns usually appear as painless, depressed, discoloured areas, with central necrosis and minimal bleeding. The presence of surface burns does not accurately predict the extent and severity of possible internal injuries, as skin with high resistance will deliver electrical energy to deeper tissues with lower resistance (7).

Arc burns

Current sparks arise between objects that are electrically charged with significantly different potentials and are not in direct contact with each other, usually a highly charged source and a ground. When an electrical arc passes from an object of high to low resistance, then it creates a high temperature pathway, which can reach 2500-5000° C, resulting in deep thermal burns at the contact site with the source and at the ground contact area, which is not always the feet. These areas usually present a dry, insensitive parchment centre and an adjacent edge of congestion around them. The internal pathway taken by the arc can be established based on the location of these surface wounds. In addition to high-voltage injuries from direct current along the arc pathway, arcs can also cause flash and flame burns, so multiple degrees of burns of varying appearance and severity may be noticed. Arcs do not appear in low-voltage injuries (7).

Flash burns

Flash burns are thermal burns produced by heat from a nearby electrical arc that can reach upwards of 5000° C and that does not enter the human body. Flash burns may extend over a large area of the body, resulting in diffuse but usually only partial-thickness burns. In this case, there is no internal electrical component (7).

Flame burns

Flame electrical burns are direct burns produced by ignition of clothing or nearby objects due to both electrothermal and arcing currents. These cause thermal burns similar to other flame burns (7).

Low-voltage burns

Low-voltage burns are similar to ordinary thermal burns and range from local erythema to full-thickness burns. Low-voltage exposure require several seconds of contact to cause skin burns, sometimes reaching current levels high enough to determine ventricular fibrillation before causing any significant skin damage. Direct contact burns may occur only if the circuit through the person was prolonged for more than a few seconds (7).

Low-voltage current determines both direct injury and thermal injuries, most often due to the heating effect of electricity turning a ring, wristwatch, bracelet or necklace incandescent resulting in a deep circumferential thermal burn. These burns are managed in the same way as other thermal burns. The mechanics and the persons working on automobiles are at greatest risk for this kind of injury, as automotive electrical systems are the most common source of low-voltage and high-amperage electricity. Low-voltage AC injury is usually encountered at the points of contact, although with prolonged contact, tissue damage may extend into profound tissues with little lateral extension as seen in high-voltage wounds. These wounds are usually treated by excision to viable tissue and appropriate skin coverage based on wound depth and location (10).

Direct contact electrical burns

Contact burns usually have a pattern from the contacted item (branding) and may appear similar to flash burns. Current flowing directly through the body will heat the tissue causing electrothermal burns, both to the surface of the skin as well as to deeper tissues, according to their resistance. Mostly, it causes lesions at the source contact point and at the ground contact point (7).

Pediatric oral burns

These are most commonly found in children younger than 4-6 years who bite, chew or suck on a household electrical cord and are the most common type of serious electrical burn in young children. These burns may cause facial deformities and growth problems of the teeth, jaw, and face. Burns of the oral cavity are produced by a local arc of current, passing from one side of the mouth to the other. The orbicularis oris muscle may be involved and cosmetic deformity of the lips may develop if the burn crosses the oral commissure. Significant edema may occur and within 2-3 days eschar formation.

Electrical injuries involving only the oral commissures are initially treated very conservatively, as the degree of injury is usually difficult to predict. Simple wound care is performed as an outpatient. The most serious complication is life-threatening bleeding from the labial artery, which can appear up to 2-3 weeks post injury if the labial artery is exposed when the eschar detaches. Families are instructed to digitally compress the labial artery if bleeding occurs and return to the emergency unit.

These patients should be referred for early follow-up to a burn specialist, plastic surgeon, and an oral surgeon. Following healing, rehabilitation options can vary, according to the severity of injury. Gentle stretching and the use of oral splints ensure good cosmetic and functional results in most patients, with reconstructive surgery being reserved for the remainder. Severe mircostomia is corrected by mucosal advancement flaps. Burns of the mid-portions of mouth heal very poorly and require a much more aggressive surgical approach with carefully planned reconstruction (7, 10).

Cardiovascular

The electrical exposure can damage the heart by:
- direct trauma to cardiac muscle fibers, leading to myocardial necrosis
- conduction abnormalities and cardiac dysrhythmias, such as asystole or ventricular fibrillation (VF), in addition to other arrhythmias.

Cardiac arrhythmia can occur and range from benign to fatal. High voltage or DC current is more often associated with asystole, and AC current typically causes ventricular fibrillation and sudden death. Ventricular fibrillation is the most common fatal arrhythmia, occurring in up to 60% of patients in whom the current pathway goes from one hand to the other hand. The most common abnormalities seen on an electrocardiogram (ECG) are sinus tachycardia, nonspecific ST- and T-wave changes, heart blocks, and prolongation of the QT interval. Ventricular fibrillation can appear at voltages as low as 50-120 mA, which is lower than the typical household current. One series showed cardiac arrhythmias following 41% of low-voltage electrical injuries (7, 9, 16).

Survivors of electrical shock can suffer from subsequent arrhythmias, most frequently sinus tachycardia and premature ventricular contractions (PVCs). However, long-term cardiac complications from electrical injury are rare (7, 9).

One study identified three cases of severe and long lasting ventricular arrhythmias, in which current passed through the thorax, with a delay of 8-12 hours between the exposure and the onset of symptoms (17). Nevertheless, other studies showed no risk of delayed arrhythmias in patients with initially normal ECGs, in low-voltage household exposures. Thus, after a low-voltage electrical injury, initial arrhythmia is not frequent, with often a nonspecific and transitory EKG expression; delayed arrhythmia is very rare. The authors concluded that children presenting to the emergency department after such an electrical shock, who are asymptomatic, without any risk factors for arrhythmia (wet skin, tetany, vertical pathway of the current, preexistent cardiological conditions, loss of consciousness) and with a normal initial EKG, do not require subsequent cardiac monitoring (18).

Respiratory

Electrical exposure can lead to respiratory arrest, as a result of:
- chest wall muscle paralysis from tetanic contraction, when the current pathway is over the thorax
- injury to the respiratory control center of the brain.

The lungs are a poor conductor of electricity and generally are not as susceptible to direct injury from electrical flow as other tissues with much lower resistance (7).

Renal

The acute renal failure is a deleterious outcome which can develop over the course of the patient's evolution, due to:
- acute tubular necrosis, as a result of hypovolemia from third spacing and huge volume shift
- rhabdomyolysis that results from massive tissue necrosis (9).

Digestive

Depending on the electrical resistance encountered at different levels of the human body, current flowing through narrow parts will be able to generate more heat and less dissipation. Therefore, fingers, hands, forearms, feet and legs can sometimes be totally destroyed, while the trunk dissipates long enough electricity to prevent damage to the viscera, except when entry and exit areas are present on the abdomen or chest. In these events, can be seen full-thickness wounds of the abdominal wall, including the peritoneum and even damaging the abdominal viscera, such as gastrocutaneous fistula, duodenocutaneous fistula or bowel perforation (19-21).

Neurologic

Electrical exposures can lead to CNS or spinal acute neurologic deficits, such as transient confusion, amnesia, seizure, impaired recall of events or even frank loss of consciousness, due to:
- direct current
- blunt trauma
- burns
- respiratory arrest as a result of impairment of the respiratory control centre of the brainstem.

Unless a patient is completely lucid with full recollection of the events, initial cervical spine immobilization is recommended.

Electrical currents cause acute muscle tetany at relatively low strengths and frequencies, like those found in most households. Muscle tetany determines victims to grasp the source, thereby prolonging contact time, and can also paralyze respiratory muscles leading to asphyxiation (7). The "locking-on" phenomenon refers to a refractory state of neuromuscular stimulation with tetanic contractions that prevents the patient's hand to release the source (9).

Further long-term neurologic complications can also appear, such as:
- seizures
- peripheral nerve damage
- delayed spinal cord syndromes
- psychiatric problems, from depression to aggressive behaviour (7).

21

ENT/ocular/head

The head is a common area of entry for high-voltage electrical exposures. The cephalic extremity injuries can be represented by:
- facial burns
- cervical spine injury
- perforated tympanic membranes; approximately two thirds of victims struck by lightning have ruptured eardrums.
- within days of the initial injury or years later (usually months), approximately 6% of the patients develop cataracts, with increasing frequency if the flow travels close to the eyes
- fixed and dilated or asymmetric pupils, due to autonomic dysfunction; this observation should not be used as a reason to stop resuscitation (7, 9).

Musculoskeletal

Electrical exposures can determine acute musculoskeletal injuries, such as:
- fractures from either severe muscle contractions or as a result of falls, more frequently encountered in upper limb long bones and in vertebrae
- rhabdomyolisis and subsequent renal failure, as a result of massive muscle damage
- compartment syndrome from burns, especially circumferential burns of the chest and extremities. In case of suspicion of a compartment syndrome, then palpation of extremity and distal neurologic, vascular, and motor examination should be performed. In these events, compartment pressure can be measured and early fasciotomy with aggressive debridement can prevent worsening evolution and subsequent limb amputation (7, 9).

Chapter 3 Diagnosis & assessment of electrical lesions

For a complete and accurate assessment of electrical lesions, a series of diagnostic steps are extremely important:
- history
- characteristics of the electrical exposure: voltage and the type of current
- age, gender, biological status, patient's comorbidities
- thorough physical examination
- laboratory and imaging studies.

At first appearance is the skin damage, which is typical for the electrical lesions and requires careful examination, for identifying the areas of contact (entry and exit points of the current), as well as the burn wounds. In case of high-voltage electrical injuries, the flow travels from the point of contact, deep through the tissues, and leaves the body through the exit point (ground). These types of injuries can lead to major and unapparent tissue damage, which is often underestimated (12).

Usually, the electric shock causes deep burns at the contact areas. Still, the depth of any burn injury is not always obvious from the beginning. A lot of imaging methods have been proposed to predict the depth of the injury soon after injury (ultrasound, intravenous fluoresceine), but none has been proved to be as reliable as clinical serial examination of the wound over time, made by an experienced burn surgeon. The final depth and consequently the degree of the burn injury typically become obvious 48 to 72 hours after aggression. Thus, the depth of the burn can be estimated according to classical clinical findings, as illustrated in Table 4 (12):

Table 4: Typical examination findings according to burn depth

Depth of burn	Symptoms	Signs
First degree	Pain	Erythema, epidermal slough 1-4 days later
Second degree	Pain	Blisters, erythema, tenderness, good capillary refill
Third degree	+/_ Pain	Insensate, leathery, thrombosed vessels, no capillary refill, +/_ blisters

The accurate assessment of the extent of tissue damage is rather difficult. The percentage of burned body surface area roughly underestimates the injury to underlying tissue. High-voltage electrical burns may appear as simple depressed and circumscribed marks. In contrast, fatal electrocution may even take place without any visible skin burns, in case of a large contact area. The extent of visible burns may not correlate to any other complications or sequelae. In contrast to ordinary thermal burns, deposition of metallic iron and copper is found on the epidermis after electrical injuries, as electrolysis occurs in the extracellular fluid matrix of the skin. Therefore, these metal condensations can produce a black and specific coating of the skin, resembling an eschar and designating the electrical contact areas (11).

In practice, clinical determination of profound tissue viability and the extent of deep tissue necrosis are based on inspection and the demonstration of muscle contractility. So far, there are no other diagnostic tests available to accurately assess the degree and the extent of tissue damage in the early phase following electrical injuries. However, multiple diagnostic methods have been proposed and investigated, to speed up the process of identifying the extent of deep tissue necrosis, such as (10, 11):

- Serial measurement of skin temperature
- Muscle perfusion scintigraphy; radionuclide scanning with xenon-133 and technetium pyrophosphate has been shown to be accurate predictors of tissue damage, but did not decrease hospital stay or number of staged operations required
- Magnetic resonance imaging (MRI), which provides poor sensitivity for assessment of muscle damage in non-perfused areas
- Gadolinium-enhanced MR imaging demonstrates potential viability in zones of tissue edema and good correlation with histopathology. While very sensitive and specific, diagnostic scans usually add little to direct clinical evaluation and produce logistical problems.
- Angiography, which does not provide information on tissue viability, but demonstrates the absence of tissue perfusion, and may lead to an early indication of limb amputation (11). Nevertheless, for all practical purposes, the use of the aforementioned techniques is expensive and unnecessary (10).

Before tissue necrosis become apparent, the physiologic damaging effects to the patient may develop almost irreversible, without proper and immediate treatment. In patients with suspected electrical injuries, a series of parameters must be addressed early, because the real extent of such injuries reveals only over time (12):

- myonecrosis with severe myoglobinemia, leading to acute renal failure
- soft tissue damage in the extremities, leading to compartment syndrome
- electrolyte abnormalities and cardiac injury, leading to fatal arrhythmias
- respiratory muscle paralysis, requiring pulmonary support.

Patients have to be carefully and particularly evaluated for skeletal injuries, as a lot of electrocuted victims have myotonic contractions or fall from a height. Distinct attention should be addressed toward the neck region, because occult cervical fractures can cause devastating spinal cord lesions (12).

Electrical function of the heart should be evaluated by an **initial ECG and subsequent cardiac rhythm monitoring** for the first 24-48 hours after injury. The duration of monitoring depends on the circumstances of the electrical shock; any patients with chest pain, arrhythmia, abnormal initial ECG, cardiac arrest, loss of consciousness, transthoracic conduction, or history of cardiac disease should undergo monitoring. Therefore, no definitive guidelines are available on duration of cardiac monitoring, but patients are unlikely to develop significant arrhythmias after 24-48 hours if they have no other significant injuries. On the other hand, several large reviews have not identified risk of delayed arrhythmia among patients with low-voltage electrical exposure and no arrhythmia upon initial presentation. One such review of 196 exposures concludes that admission for cardiac monitoring is not indicated for such patients (22). Several studies have shown that low-voltage (household) exposures in patients with no cardiac complaints and a normal initial ECG can be safely discharged (23). It is unclear how this applies to patients with preexisting heart disease. In the paediatric population, healthy children presenting household current exposures and without water contact can be safely discharged if they are asymptomatic, without arrhythmia or cardiac arrest and have no other injuries requiring admission (7, 18, 24).

The following **laboratory tests** are indicated in all patients with more than a trivial electrical exposure (7, 9):
  - Complete blood cell count
  - Glucose level
  - Serum electrolyte levels
  - Liver function tests
  - Blood urea nitrogen and creatinine, due to high risk of rhabdomyolysis and myoglobinuria in electrical injuries
  - Urinalysis: specific gravity, pH, hematuria, and urine myoglobin if urinalysis is positive for hemoglobin
  - Serum myoglobin, if urine is positive for myoglobin
  - Arterial blood gas and pulse oximetry for patients who require ventilatory support, those with suspected smoke inhalation or those with severe rhabdo-myolysis needing urine alkalinization therapy
  - Creatine kinase (CK) levels. This level may be extremely elevated in electrocuted patients with massive muscle damage from high-voltage injuries. Some evidence suggests that initial CK levels may help predict which patients could benefit from early fasciotomy to prevent subsequent amputations (25). CK-MB subfractions are also often elevated in electrical injuries, but their significance in the framework of electrical exposures is not well known. If possible, CK-MB fractions and troponin should be checked if the current pathway involved the thorax, if the patient has any signs of ischemia or arrhythmia on ECG, or if the patient has specific complaints of chest pain.

Some studies have suggested that CK and CK-MB levels are poor indicators of myocardial injury in the absence of ECG signs of myocardial injury, especially in the presence of significant skeletal muscle damage (10).

- Further, more severely injured patients who require surgery may need: blood typing or cross matching, prothrombin time, and activated partial thromboplastin time studies.

One retrospective review revealed a decision and simple rule for clinical identification of patients predisposed to rhabdomyolysis. Multivariate modeling highlighted that high-voltage injuries, prehospital cardiac arrest, full-thickness burns, and compartment syndrome were highly associated with myoglobinuria. Defining "positive" as the presence of minimum two of these findings has a sensitivity of 96% and a negative predictive value of 99% (7, 26)

The **imaging studies** are indicated according to type of electrical exposure, blunt trauma, patient complaints, altered mental status, cardiac or respiratory arrest (7, 9):

- Chest radiography, to any patient with cardiac or respiratory arrest, dyspnoea, chest pain, hypoxia, CPR at the scene, or fall/blunt trauma
- Head computed tomography, to any patient with altered mental status, significant traumatic mechanism, seizure, loss of consciousness, or focal neurologic deficits
- Cervical spine and pelvis radiographs, to any patient with loss of consciousness or with significant trauma, which should be cervical spine immobilized and imaged accordingly. Patients with focal neurologic deficits or evidence of spinal cord injury should undergo full spinal imaging. Appropriate extremity films should also be obtained in patients with obvious extremity injuries.
- CT and ultrasonography, which are further imaging studies to assess the range and extent of internal injuries, according to availability, the severity of trauma and the pathway of the current exposure.

A special attention should be directed to the possible development of increased myofascial compartment pressures, as a result of vascular ischemia and muscle edema, especially in high-voltage injuries. If this is anticipated, each compartment must be checked and measured. Surgical decompression is usually necessary, if signs and symptoms of compartment syndrome develop. The defining sign of compartment syndrome is pain with passive motion in the compartment containing the muscle groups which are responsible for that motion. Characteristically, the pain is unrelenting and may occur without proportional connection to the visible injury. Patients can also complain of paresthesia, hypoesthesia, or decreased motor function. Finally, loss of pulses is a very late sign occurring in compartment syndrome (9, 27).

The electrical burn lesion should be seen as a constantly evolving lesion, even more than other thermal burn. Especially in high-voltage exposures, the most commonly seen evolution is to burn deepening. Serial debridements, decompression fasciotomy or even amputation are frequently necessary in cases of extensive tissue damage. The massive release of myoglobin from the damaged muscle can lead to myoglobinuric acute renal failure. Vascular damage from the electrical flow may become evident at any time following exposure. Pulses and capillary refill should be checked and documented in all extremities, and neurovascular exams should be repeated frequently. Because the arteries are a high-flow vascular system, heat may be dissipated fairly well and cause little apparent initial damage, but result in subsequent damage. On the other hand, the veins are a low-flow vascular system, which allows the electrical flow to cause a more rapid heating of the blood and to produce thrombosis. Therefore, an extremity may initially appear edematous. In case of severe electrical injuries, the entire extremity can appear mummified when all tissue elements, including the arteries, suffer from coagulation necrosis. Damage to the vessel wall at the time of the injury may also result in delayed thrombosis and hemorrhage, especially in the small muscle arteries. This ongoing vascular damage can cause a partial-thickness burn to develop into a full-thickness burn as the vascular supply to the area diminishes. Progressive deterioration of muscles due to vascular ischemia downstream from damaged vessels can usually require repeated and deep surgical debridements (27).

Especially in high-voltage exposures, a series of additional neurological disorders may occur, such as (27):

- loss of consciousness, usually transient in the absence of a significant concomitant head injury
- prolonged coma with eventual recovery
- confusion
- flat affect
- difficulty with short-term memory and concentration
- seizure due to electrical injury to the central nervous system (CNS), hypoxia and traumatic CNS injury, either as an isolated event or as part of a new-onset seizure disorder
- lower extremity weakness is commonly undiagnosed until ambulation is attempted.

Neurologic symptoms may improve, but long-term disability is common. In high-voltage exposures, spinal cord injury can result from fractures or from ligamentous disruption of the cervical, thoracic, or lumbar spine (27).

Chapter 4 Treatment guidelines after electrical aggression

First aid (prehospital care)

In the first instance, place safety should be ensured, without imminent threat to bystanders or responders in attempting to pull the victim out from the electrical source. In case of high-voltage exposures, the source voltage should be turned off before rescue workers enter the scene.

After ensuring place safety, rescuers should approach victims of electrical injuries as both trauma and cardiac patients. Airway, breathing, circulation, and inline immobilization of the spine should be accomplished as an integral part of primary care. Patients may need basic or advanced cardiac life support and should undergo spinal immobilization as indicated by the mechanism of injury. Hidden injuries should also be suspected and clinically evaluated.

Given that injuries may be limited to a ventricular arrhythmia or respiratory muscle paralysis, aggressive and prolonged CPR should be initiated in the field for all electrical injury victims, taking into account that they are likely to be younger with fewer comorbidities and have better prognosis after prolonged CPR (7, 9).

Medical therapy

As previously stated, patients with electrical injury should be initially evaluated and accordingly treated as a trauma patient (28). Intravenous access, cardiac monitoring, and measurement of oxygen saturation should be started during the primary survey, in all patients with electrical injuries; furthermore, central access should be taken into account in any patient with significant trauma, large burns, cardiac or respiratory arrest, or loss of consciousness (7, 9).

Electrically injured patients should be stabilized and provided airway and circulatory support, according to emergency cardiovascular and trauma care protocols. Airway protection and oxygen should be provided for any patient with severe hypoxia, facial and oral burns, loss of consciousness and inability to protect airway, or respiratory distress (7).

All patients should be monitored during transport and in the emergency unit. Rather than a policy of more prolonged cardiac monitoring for all patients, a selective protocol makes most efficient use of expensive medical resources, without patient risk. Thus, indications for cardiac monitoring are as follows:
- Documented cardiac arrest
- Cardiac arrhythmia on transport or in ER
- Abnormal EKG in ER (other than sinus brady- or tachycardia)
- Burn size or patient age would require monitoring (10).

Cervical spine immobilization with or without spinal immobilization is also required, according to the mechanism of electrical injury and neurologic examination. Besides, primary survey should assess for additional traumatic injuries such as pneumothorax, peritonitis, or skeletal fractures (7).

Maybe more than in other thermal injuries, **fluid replacement** is the most important part of the initial resuscitation, as electrical injuries cause massive fluid shifts with extensive tissue damage and acidosis. Therefore, monitoring a patient's hemodynamics is extremely important. Usually, a Foley catheter is used in monitoring urine output and, therefore, tissue perfusion.

The target for initial fluid resuscitation is done by urine output greater than 0.5 cc/kg/h if no signs of myoglobinuria are present and preferably greater than 1 cc/kg/h if myoglobinuria is present. Since lightning burns are usually superficial, using a standard formula for burns, such as the Parkland formula, may be helpful (9).

Maybe the most widely used formula today in burn shock resuscitation, the **Parkland formula** recommends **4 mL of Ringer's lactate/kg/% TBSA** (total body surface area) burned in the first 24 hours, an isotonic balanced saline solution, with one-half of that amount administered in the first 8 hours after the exposure (29).

However, the unpredictable nature and extent of electrical injuries make difficult to assess the volume of tissue damage and to estimate fluid deficits. Many authors increase fluid replacement after an electrical injury, up to 2-3 times over the volume calculated based on the Parkland formula, depending on the total surface area potentially involved. The urinary output is a particularly valuable indicator of hemodynamic status and kidney function. Regular and constant adjustments of the fluid resuscitation should be practiced, according to hourly urine output. Thus, fluid rates should decrease or increase to maintain urine output of 0.5-1 cc/kg/h (9).

Hematuria or dark urine prompts the need for more aggressive therapy to prevent myoglobin-induced tubular necrosis (9). The appearance of pigmented (darker than light pink) urine in an electrical injured patient indicates significant muscle damage. Myoglobin and hemoglobin pigments can lead to acute renal failure and must be cleared promptly. While their low levels are of little clinical concern, highly evident urinary pigmentation requires fast and dynamic response, in order to minimize renal tubular obstruction. The urine aspect is too sensitive for both pigments and hematuria to serve as a guide for treatment. The assessment of the serum to distinguish between myoglobin and hemoglobin depends on the fact that the smaller myoglobin complex is cleared by the kidney at a threshold below visibility, while hemoglobin as a polymer is bound to albumin, and has a much higher renal threshold. However, differentiating between the two is of little clinical importance, as both require prompt clearance and must be accordingly managed (10).

Urine with a color darker than light pink is promptly treated with fluids (initiating diuresis) and bicarbonate. Ringer's lactate is administered at a rate sufficient to maintain an efficient urinary output and to grossly clear the urine of pigment. **Bicarbonate** is administered at 1-2 mEq/kg and **mannitol** at 1 gram per kilogram body weight, in order to promote and to maintain osmotic diuresis. Mannitol is an osmotic diuretic that is not metabolized significantly and that passes through glomerulus without being reabsorbed by the kidney. Bicarbonate can be given with the initial fluid bolus, in situation of very extensive electrical injuries, when acidosis and myoglobinuria are anticipated Bicarbonate treats the underlying acidosis and alkalinizes the urine, making myoglobin more soluble. The target is a urine output up to 2-3 mL/kg/h, with a urine pH greater than 6.5. The rationale of this protocol is to create a rapid, osmotic diuresis with initial alkalinization to minimize pigment precipitation in the renal tubules. The required urinary output is usually very high for several hours following injury, followed by significant reduction in urine requirements, as venous return from the injured part to the central circulation is thrombosed (7, 9, 10).

Additional diuretics may be administered. Loop diuretics are not as efficient as mannitol. Acetazolamide is the recognized drug of choice because it also alkalinizes the urine. However, this diuresis should be practiced with extreme caution to avoid hyperosmotic hypoalbuminemia (9, 10).

Electrical burn management should also require tetanus immunization as indicated, wound care, measurement of compartment pressures as indicated, and it may include early fasciotomy. Extremities with severe electrical injuries should be splinted in a functional position after careful documentation of full neurovascular examination and appropriate treatment (7).

The infection risk is major in electrical injuries, due to damage of natural defence barrier represented by the skin, as well as to presence of ischemic and devitalized deep tissues. Consequently, the therapeutic protocol stipulates the immediate administration of a treatment with broad spectrum antibiotics or with an association of antibiotics (27).

Patients exposed to low-voltage electrical sources that are otherwise absolutely asymptomatic and with a normal physical examination can usually be discharged from the emergency department. Patients with minor burns or mild symptoms can be observed for several hours and discharged if their symptoms resolve and they do not have elevated CK or myoglobinuria. Patients should be cautioned about the possible long-term neurologic or ocular complications of electrical injuries, and have follow-up available as required. On the other hand, inpatient care and prompt treatment are required for all patients with anything other than minor low-voltage injuries. Burn and trauma care, preferably at a specialized center, should be initiated as early as possible. Any patients with cardiac arrest, loss of consciousness, abnormal ECG, hypoxia, chest pain, dysrhythmias, and significant burns or traumatic injuries must be admitted. All patients with a history of exposure to high-voltage electricity and patients with significant burns should be transferred to a specialized burn center for further inpatient treatment and rehabilitation (7).

In a pregnant patient, the risks of electrical injury to the fetus are not really known. Pregnant women who are involved in electrical injuries should undergo a careful and complete examination for traumatic injuries and obstetrical consultation. Pregnant women should be admitted for electrical burn management and fetal monitoring in any cases of severe electrical injuries, high-voltage exposures, or minor electrical injuries with significant trauma (7).

Surgical therapy

The electrical lesions can present early surgical indication for two reasons:
- Prolonged ischemia and massive necrosis of the deep tissues can induce profound acidosis and myoglobinuria, which cannot be treated by common medical methods of resuscitation. These situations may require large incisions in emergency, with fasciotomies, extensive debridements and even amputation.
- More often, prevention and treatment of compartment syndrome that develops following tissue edema. Careful monitoring is mandatory in affected extremity, to detect signs of peripheral neuropathy compression. The finding of functional deficit of median or (rarely) ulnar nerves in the affected hand is an indication for immediate nerve decompression at the wrist (opening of carpal and Guyon channels). If immediate decompression or surgical debridement is unnecessary for the moment, then definitive surgery can be practiced between 3 and 5 days after the exposure, before producing bacterial contamination and after delimitation of tissue necrosis (30, 31). Sometimes special measures can be applied, such as vascular grafts to replace thrombosed and compromised arteries, or even free emergency transfers (32, 33), but caution is required, because these aggressive surgical measures can increase morbidity and prolong patient recovery. A well-adapted prosthesis can be more functional than an insensitive and weak hand or foot (10).

Fasciotomy of a burned extremity may be urgently required in high-voltage injuries or prolonged low-voltage injuries, as aggressive early intervention via fasciotomy can prevent subsequent limb amputation (7). Thus, a low threshold for fasciotomy is always indicated, because an early fasciotomy may prevent limb ischemia and also may prevent or limit the extent of amputation. The burn surgeon should take account that the external appearance of an electrical burn may underestimate the degree of underlying deep tissue destruction. The liberal indications for fasciotomy cannot be overemphasized because the morbidity associated with a failure to perform a strictly required fasciotomy by far exceeds that caused by the procedure itself. The most important contraindication would be the failure to promptly and correctly manage more severely life-threatening electrical injuries or complications of electrical shock, or the failure to adequately resuscitate the patient prior to surgical intervention, which should be done after aggressive resuscitation has reversed shock, assured oxygen delivery, restored circulating volume, and reestablished end-organ perfusion (9).

Therefore, the functional outcome of an electrical burn lesion is inversely proportional to the time elapsed before the beginning of the reconstructive interventions. According to characteristics of the electrical lesions, tissue damage leads to vascular thrombosis and skin and muscle necrosis. The optimal management of these wounds has evolved to initial debridement, decompression (fasciotomy), aggressive serial deep tissue debridement and early skin coverage with the aim of preserving vital structures (9, 28).

The excisions until viable tissues or even the amputations performed in emergency intend to limit the extension of the ischemic lesions and the resorption of cell degradation products. The increase of CK is not an indicative factor itself in performing re-excisions but orients the therapeutic approach, the utilization of the dialysis when the values do not decrease by medical therapy for renal support and the forcing of diuresis is required. The normalization of CK indicates the time when reconstructive surgery can begin for covering of the defects resulted as a consequence of the excisions. The level of the leukocytes represents both a prognostic factor and an indicative factor for the re-excision of the ischemic areas. An increased level under antibiotic therapy signifies either an incomplete excision or the wound infection with bacteria resistant to the antibiotics that have been used (27).

Fasciotomy serves a dual role in the management of electrical injuries, as both a therapeutic tool and a diagnostic tool in assessing the extent of muscular necrosis. The defining feature of electrical lesion is the fact that a burn with a relatively small surface area may hide and denote massive tissue destruction beneath. Therefore, any swelling or signs of impaired circulation should be early and aggressively evaluated and managed. Impaired circulation to extremities after burn injury may be the result of constrictive burn eschar, which usually is circumferential and of full thickness, as well as the result of compartment syndrome, which is caused by edematous muscles. Any suspicious extremity must be examined in the operating room by removing burn eschar initially, followed by fasciotomy and debridement as indicated (9).

Reconstructive options for coverage of electrical burn wounds encompass the total range of plastic reconstructive procedures: delayed closure, skin grafts, locoregional flaps, myocutaneous, fasciocutaneous, muscle flaps and free tissue transfer. Split thickness skin graft may serve as an intermediate biological cover or as a definitive procedure. Limb salvage with functional preservation of vital structures should always be attempted and may require revascularization using segmental vein grafts or nervous reconstruction using segmental nerve grafting. Pedicled flaps should be considered in cases of suspected arterial compromise. In severe cases, early amputation remains the only safe alternative (9, 11).

Chapter 5 Complications of electrical lesions

The primary early complications of electrical lesions include (9, 10, 27):
- renal damage
- wound infection and sepsis, managed in the standard approach
- cardiac injury, recognized and treated on admission
- neurological deficits, that may be present on admission or may develop in days to weeks after injury
- ocular manifestations
- compartment syndrome, which can be avoided through fasciotomies, debridements or carpal tunnel release
- tissue loss and major amputations, common in severe high-voltage injuries and needing subsequent extensive rehabilitation.
- stress ulcer, the most usual gastrointestinal complication after burn ileus
- abdominal injuries from ischemia, vascular damage, burns, or associated blunt trauma, which may be initially neglected.

Pneumonia, sepsis, and multisystem organ failure are the most common causes of hospital mortality. Acute renal failure and sepsis can be prevented and managed by adequate fluid resuscitation to maintain an efficient urinary output and by rapid removal of necrotic burn tissue. In present, the incidence of acute myoglobinuric renal failure has lowered, as a result of the aggressive alkalinized fluid resuscitation (27).

Another significant complication after electrical flow is limb dysfunction by complex regional pain syndrome (CRPS), which can be improved through early, sustained physical and occupational therapy (9).

Cataract development represents the most frequent ocular complication due to electrical injury, although ocular electrical determinations may involve all portions of the eye (including iritis, macular holes, and central retinal artery occlusion). The exact pathophysiology remains unknown, but ocular changes may concern as high as 5–20% of patients with true electrical burns. Contact points of the head, neck and upper trunk show a higher risk for cataract formation, although some reports exhibited a high rate of bilaterality and no relation with voltage, path of the electrical flow or location of entry points. Cataract may also occur without injury to the head and may appear between 3 weeks and even 11 years after injury. Common initial complaints are blurred vision or diminished visual acuity. In such cases, visual acuity and fundoscopic examination should be performed in initial emergency assessment. Almost half of the patient presenting cataract needed surgical therapy, the result of which were constantly favourable (10, 11, 27, 34-37).

Neurological complications show a wide diversity and may occur either early or late (up to 2 years after exposure). Neurological damage in patients without evidence of spinal injury may follow two patterns:

- immediate damage, developing within hours of the electrical exposure through symptoms of weakness and paresthesias. Lower extremity findings are more frequent than upper extremity findings. These patients present a good prognosis for partial or complete recovery.

- delayed neurological damage, occurring from days to years after the exposure. The neuromuscular defects include paralysis, seizure, Guillain–Barré syndrome, transverse myelitis or amyotrophic lateral sclerosis. Motor findings predominate. Sensory findings are also present, but they may be irregular and may not fit the motor levels. Although recovery is reported, the prognosis is usually poor (10, 27).

Approximately two thirds of patients with high-voltage injury developed immediate central or peripheral neurological symptoms, loss of consciousness being the predominant symptom. The most common peripheral neurological defect is a peripheral neuropathy, with weakness being the most usually found clinical finding. In general, spasticity is more frequent than flaccidity, function is affected more than sensation, and resolution of early-onset neurological deficits is much better than for late onset. The primary autonomic complex complication is sympathetic overactivity with changes in bowel habits, urinary and sexual functions. Although the exact mechanism of nerve injury has not been explained, both direct injury by electrical current and/or a vascular cause are possible mechanisms. A full neurological examination should be performed in initial emergency presentation. Long-term follow-up with neuromuscular examinations and electrodiagnostic evaluation are an important part of patient management. To date, prognosis or assessment of the extent of neurological damage hasn't been accurately accomplished through imaging studies, including angiography and MR imaging (10, 11, 38, 39).

Very often, neuropsychological status is altered following electrical shock. Typical complaints are related to physical, cognitive, and emotional changes. These consequences could not be directly attributed to physical manifestations of injury, and are similar to problems associated with prolonged stress, sleep deprivation, or after blunt head injury. Whilst the development of transient and progressive neuropsychiatric complications after electrical exposure is possible and not controversial, the effective specific mechanisms of electrical injury are difficult to clearly establish. Other concomitant factors can influence systematic evaluation, such as the posttraumatic stress disorder, the disposition of the patient and the grief reaction to disfigurement or extremity loss. Therefore, long-term neuropsychiatric complications include: depression, anxiety, inability to continue in the same profession, aggressive behavior, and suicide. Early involvement of an experienced psychiatrist is important in assessing long-term needs and taking part in elaboration of a therapy plan (10, 11, 27, 40-42).

Chapter 6 Prognosis & prevention of electrical lesions

Following low-voltage exposures, for patients without significant burns, prolonged consciousness, respiratory or cardiac arrest, the prognosis for full recovery is excellent. Nevertheless, rare persistent arrhythmias may be possible. Persistence of unconsciousness determines a worse prognosis, and the complete recovery of the patient cannot be expected after 24 hours of unconsciousness. Patients who suffered low-voltage injuries with cardiac or respiratory arrest may recover completely with immediate CPR on place; however, prolonged CPR and transport time may cause neurological deficits, as well as permanent brain damage.

Electrical burns and traumatic injuries continue to determine the majority of the morbidity and mortality, which are highly influenced by the properties and characteristics of the particular electrical flow involved in each patient. Thereby, high-voltage and prolonged exposures commonly result in serious burns and blunt trauma. Patients are at high risk of sepsis, myoglobinuria and renal failure, and burns are usually more severe and extensive than they initially appeared in the emergency unit, needing surgical aggressive treatment (7)

However, even massive electrical burns have good chances of survival, and overall mortality is estimated to be 3-15%. Flash burns have a better prognosis than arc or conductive burns (7, 43).

Final outcome and prognosis are determined by the location and extent of electrical lesions, the development of complications and the functional results. Recent advances in modern ICU care, fluid resuscitation, nutritional support, and surgical aggressive techniques, along with the development of new skin substitutes, have significantly ameliorated the outcomes and prognosis (9). However, substantial morbidity from traumatic injuries and electrical burns, as well as rates of amputation still remains relatively high (7).

Since most electrical injuries are preventable, the most important factors for prevention management and prognosis improvement are patient education and compliance to safety measures both at home and at work (9, 28).

Prevention of high-voltage electrical exposures requires constantly public education about potential hazards, and targeted education to people in construction activities, those using cranes and lifts, or those exposed to the outermost danger of overhead power lines. Studies revealed especially high rates of severe electrical injuries in cable splicers, electricians, line workers, and substation operators. Therefore, prevention strategies and occupational safety measures should be oriented toward these high-risk occupations. Also, prevention of less dangerous household exposures requires general public education about child protection, outlet covers, and appliance safety. Moreover, appliances that can produce an electrical shock should not be used until professionally repaired (7, 44).

Chapter 7 Skeletal injuries due to electrical aggression

In terms of pathophysiology, clinical and therapeutic approach, the osteoarticular injuries represent a distinct and specific category, which is often overlooked, with deleterious effects and subsequent unfavorable complaints.

Throughout the human body, the electrical flow would be theoretically distributed according to different tissue resistances, with the highest resistance generating the most heat. Nevertheless, in the animal model, the body acts as a single uniform resistance rather than a congregation of different resistances and it comports oneself as a volume conductor. Deep tissues seem to retain heat so that the peri-osseous tissues often undergo a more severe damage than superficial tissue, especially between two adiacent bones, such as in the forearm (radius–ulna) and in the leg (tibia–fibula). Besides, the associated macro- and microscopic vascular injuries seem to develop almost immediately and are not reversible. Electrical flow produces tissue injuries directly, by heating effect, as well as by indirect destruction of cells, which seems to be particularly important for nervous system cells, as their damage cannot be explained by heating alone. Human cells have the potential for membrane breakdown with the passage of high voltage alternating current and disruption of cell membranes is one of the mechanisms by which cell damage can occur, as cell membranes are electrically charged and maintain their integrity with a sodium-potassium-ATPase pump functioning at −90 millivolts direct current. This process of electroporation of cellular membranes may explain the injury not apparently caused by heat (10). On the other hand, as previously shown, the osseous tissue presents the lowest resistance and the highest conductance to electrical flow and consequently the bones are the least electrically injured though heating action.

Skeletal injuries following electrical exposures are rather uncommon. The pathophysiology of skeletal lesions implies indirectly damage of the osseous tissues through additional trauma, in contrast to direct injury of the soft tissues through electrical energy. The usual cause of skeletal injury after electrocution is a fall due to the electrical shock. Also, fractures following electroconvulsive therapy (ECT) for psychiatric patients are a well-known complication described in literature, but skeletal injuries as a result of accidental electrical flow are very unusual (14, 51, 52). Thus, fractures or dislocations can result from tetanic muscular contractions (52). The most frequently affected level after electro-convulsive therapy (ECT) was a vertebra, in 40% of all fractures (53). ECT therapy represents the major cause of most bilateral femoral neck fractures (52) and the fractures of the lower limbs represent 28% of all fractures due to ECT, all of them being femoral neck fractures (53).

Therefore, a series of fractures and dislocations can occur following electrical injury, as a result of two distinct pathophysiologic mechanisms:
- secondary falls associated with electrical shock

- forceful muscle contractions, due to direct muscle electrical stimulation or to seizures caused by electrical exposures (54).

These are mostly seen in the shoulder, wrists, femurs and the spine, and may require aggressive surgical treatment through open reduction and internal fixation (11, 45-48). Generally, fractures after electrocution occur in places with significant and bulky muscular bodies, such as spine, hip and shoulder.

The performed review of literature has revealed several cases of fracture after accidental electrical injuries, only 22 cases being identified in a review published in 2014 (14), at the following sites:
- vertebrae (12, 14);
- neck of femur (14, 51-55);
- shoulder: scapula and proximal humerus (14, 45, 56-64);
- forearm: Colles, Galeazzi, greenstick and distal radius (14, 46, 65-67).

These fractures appear as a result of musculoskeletal contractions, which may develop even at low-voltage exposures (48, 59, 67). The threshold for tetanic muscle contractions from direct current is approximately 50 V. Muscular contractions may result from contact with a direct current of at least 20 mA or with an alternating current of 10 mA (51).

Delay in diagnostic of fractures after electrocution may be of days, weeks or even months after injury (1, 3, 54), taking into account that there is no direct trauma to the musculoskeletal system, the fractures being caused by strong tetanic muscular contractions. Local pain and swelling can be initially attributed to deep muscle contractions and to the damage to the soft tissues. Therefore, a detailed and complete physical examination of the musculoskeletal system should be practiced in these patients in the emergency unit, especially when they complain of musculoskeletal damages. X-ray films are often unnecessary in awake and cooperative patients, with no significant pain and tenderness, full active range of motion of the joints, and good function. In the unconscious or uncooperative patient, x-ray films of the shoulders, spine, and pelvis are recommended, especially if such structures were in the pathway of the electric current (51).

In general, the delay in diagnosis and further treatment of fractures after electrocution may be related to:
- a delay in presentation of the patient
- the investigation and the treatment of apparently greater comorbidities (cardiac disturbance, dermal burns, myonecrosis leading to renal failure)
- the difficulty in obtaining a clear history and physical examination on a recently electrocuted patient (14).

Especially for femoral neck fractures and in young patients, the delay in diagnosis and therapy determines common detrimental complications and unfavourable long-term outcomes:

- the progression of undisplaced fracture to a displaced fracture of femoral neck
- the risk of non-union and osteonecrosis of femoral head with functional disability, pain and degenerative joint disease (51, 52).

The therapeutic management of fractures and dislocations after electrical exposures is common and accurate, according to the principles of orthopaedic surgery and considering the other comorbidities and electrical determinations.

In high voltage exposures, electrothermic effects can lead to osteonecrosis and melting of bone tissue. On the surface of injured bone may appear grayish white and hollow osseous pearls (54).

Late sequelae of electrical injury similar to severe thermal burns include:
- major joint contractures
- limited function of the extremities (11).

Another common late skeletal complication of electrical burns is the **heterotopic calcification** in periarticular tissue of large joints, especially elbows. Causative factors may include:
- forced passive mobilization
- secondary articular bleeding
- calcium precipitation and deposition in damaged or degenerating muscle and connective tissue (11).

Unique to the electrically burned patient, **heterotopic bone formation** can occur at the cut ends of amputation stumps, in up to 80% of patients with long bone amputations, but not in patients with disarticulations or small bone amputations. Together with common formation of bone cysts in the amputation stump, these events may lead to secondary skin erosion, inflammation, and difficult adjustment of prosthesis. Thus, heterotopic ossification can be severe enough to require surgical revision of the bone end in 28% of cases. Adequate surgical therapy can be easily accomplished by opening the stump incision, excision of the soft heterotopic bone and wound closure (10, 11, 49).

Damage to developing dentition may also be detected in younger children with mouth burn, which is the most common electrical injury seen in children less than 4 years of age and which occurs from biting, chewing or sucking on a household electrical extension. This situation is recommended to be managed by an oral surgeon familiar with electrical injuries (27, 50).

Chapter 8 Osteoarticular injuries of the axial skeleton

The axial skeleton (80 bones) maintains the upright posture of the body and it consists of the following components:
- the spine/vertebral column: 7 cervical vertebrae, 12 thoracic vertebrae, 5 lumbar vertebrae, sacral and coccygeal bones
- a part of the rib cage: 12 pairs of ribs and the sternum
- the skull: 22 bones (8 cranial and 14 facial) and 7 associated bones (hyoid and auditory ossicle bones).

The axial skeleton transmits the weight from the head, the trunk, and the upper extremities down to the lower extremities at the hip joints. The bones of the spine are supported, balanced and protected by a series of ligaments and muscles, such as the erector spinae muscles. Due to important muscle coverage, prone to tetanic contractions after electrical flow, vertebral column may suffer fractures at different levels.

Vertebral fractures are more common after low-voltage and alternating current, as compared to direct current, and should be suspected in electrically injured patients with the following signs and symptoms:
- back pain
- neurologic deficits
- continuous loss of consciousness (54).

Fractures have been mentioned in literature as a possible complication of psychiatric patients exposed to electroconvulsive therapy (ECT) (51). Electric convulsive spine fractures following electroshock therapy have been reported since 1940's, with an overall fracture incidence of 6.3%. All thoracic vertebrae can be involved between T2 and T11, and the average number of fractured vertebrae among those who suffered fractures was 2.6. There was no increased tendency to fracture associated with kyphosis, scoliosis, arthritis, nuclear change or old fractures. However, osteoporosis appeared to predispose to fractures and doubled the incidence compared to other cases (68).

Multiple spine injury after electrical exposures is extremely rare. Cervical and thoracic fractures can be produced by tetanic muscle contractions leading to powerful flexion or extension of the neck and trunk. They can be suspected by the occurring of severe neck pain, even in the absence of neurologic damage, and can be detected on spinal films and CT scanning. Such neurologically intact 38-year-old patient with fracture of the spinous process of C2 and compression fractures of C5, T7 and T11, due to electrical tetanic muscle contractions, associated with 10% body surface area partial-thickness burns of the hands, forearms, right thigh and scrotum, was successfully treated by external orthopaedic stabilization in a halo-body cast for 12 weeks (54, 69).

Another 34-year-old man, who had no significant medical history and no history of remote trauma, sustained a low-voltage electrical shock, without fall or loss of consciousness. The patient had his shoulders forcefully retracted and his neck and thoracic spine hyperextended, and he complained of immediate pain in the right shoulder and midthoracic spine. He was found to have a right scapular fracture, which was conservatively managed. However, his midback pain persisted for three months after the accident, without chest or extremity pain, palpitations, dyspnoea, weakness, numbness and paresthesia. Physical examination showed stable gait, painful thoracolumbar range of motion, and diffuse tenderness to palpation of the upper thoracic spine, with point tenderness around the T4 spinous process. His detailed neurologic examination was customary. X-ray of the thoracic spine highlighted T4 compression fracture, and magnetic resonance imaging (MRI) scan of the thoracic spine confirmed the presence of a subacute T4 compression fracture, without retropulsion and without evidence to suggest pathologic fracture. There was no evidence of a burst fracture or signal change within the spinal cord. This injury was probably related to the forceful hyperextension of the thoracic spine, following the passing of the current from one arm through the midthoracic spine and scapula to the contralateral arm. The patient was referred to Interventional Radiology, but his fracture location was appreciated to be positioned too high in the thoracic spine to be managed by kyphoplasty or vertebroplasty. The patient was conservatively treated and underwent physical therapy, but unfortunately his midback pain persisted and the patient could not return to his previous level of work and physical activity. He was subsequently treated with pain medication and a thoracolumbosacral orthesis brace for support (70, 71).

Lumbar fractures following low-voltage exposures can be suspected by the occurring of persistent low back pain and tenderness, with or without neurologic deficits. The diagnosis is established by plain radiograph and CT scan. Thus, in a 62-year old electrocuted patient, with burn on the left hand, low back pain and no neurologic signs, X-ray revealed a fracture of L4 with involvement of the dorsal cortex of the corpus. CT scan highlighted a burst fracture with anterior and middle spinal column involvement, and with a small bony fragment in the spinal canal. He was treated with a plaster corset, and was mobilized one week after admission. No neurological complications occurred in evolution. Physical examination and radiographic follow-up 3 months later revealed consolidation without deformation (48, 54).

Lesions of the skull after electrical exposure are uncommon and appear especially after high-voltage injuries, often associated with very deep burns and serious brain injuries (54). Their management requires surgical approach for skull covering through complex reconstructive procedures, such as locoregional flaps or free flaps, sometimes in combination with neurosurgical reconstruction. Skin grafts are fragile and unstable in the long term; they can be applied in small defects and only if the periosteum is intact or over the granulation tissue developed after perforation or removal of the outer table (72).

Chapter 9 Osteoarticular injuries of the shoulder and upper limb

The appendicular skeleton (126 bones) is formed by:
- the pectoral girdles (shoulder girdle): clavicle and scapula
- the upper limbs
- the pelvic girdle (hip girdle or pelvis): hip or coxal bones
- the lower limbs.

Their functions are to make prehension, work and locomotion possible, and to protect the major organs of digestion, excretion and reproduction.

In electrocuted patients, shoulder region seems to be the most involved in producing fractures and dislocations, due to a series of contributing factors:
- its great joint mobility
- significant and powerful surrounding muscle and tendons, prone to violent contractures
- frequently located in electrical flow path, with hand as contact point
- may be surprised by the electric discharge in unfavourable positions.

Scapular fractures are uncommon injuries and usually caused by direct high-energy trauma. There have also been reported following cardiopulmonary resuscitation, seizures and electro-convulsive therapy. Fractures from electrical exposures usually occur when the patient falls after the accident. Nevertheless, scapula fractures as a direct result of electrical shock are very rare, with only few reported cases in the literature (56).

The scapula has multiple muscle attachments, both origins and insertions, prone to violent electric contractions. However, dislocation of the shoulder is a more frequent form of injury seen after upper limb electrocution. Significant disability has been found in patients with displaced scapular, spine and neck fractures, especially pain at rest in 50–100% and in passive or active motions. The emergency physician of a patient suffering low voltage electrical injury should have a high degree of clinical suspicion towards these injuries. These fractures can be indicated by some signs and symptoms, such as pain, bony or soft tissue tenderness and limited degree of mobility (73).

Thus, a 33-year-old patient complained of severe pain up his right arm and into his right shoulder and upper back, following an electric shock, without chest pain or palpitations, and without direct injury to the scapula. On physical examination, there were three small entry wounds at the tip of the thumb and on the radial side of the index and middle fingers. No exit wounds were noted. There were no cardiac or neurovascular alterations. He had a painful right shoulder with very low range of movement. X-ray highlighted a fracture to the blade of the right scapula. There were no associated fractures of the shoulder, which was in joint. He was admitted for cardiac monitoring and analgesia. CT scan was performed to assess the extent of the fracture and to rule out extension into the glenoid. He was discharged 24 h later with a broad arm sling and he was recommended physiotherapy exercises to mobilise the shoulder as pain allowed. At 10 days, clinical review in scapular fracture revealed a substantial periscapular haematoma, but his range of movements had greatly improved. Clinically, at 3-month review, the scapula was fully healed with no residual tenderness and a return to normal function (56).

Another 48-year-old electrician was seen three weeks after suffering an electric shock, through his right hand, while the arm was held in about 110° abduction. He immediately complained of severe pain in his right shoulder, without fall or loss of consciousness. Initially he was unable to actively move his right shoulder. X-ray performed the next day included only A-P views and apparently did not reveal any abnormality. Three weeks after the electric shock, the patient had 90° of active abduction. When the arm was abducted further passively, then a prominent lump became visible, apparently inferior to the scapular angle. True lateral radiographs were performed, to rule out a posterior dislocation. These views revealed a comminuted fracture of the scapular body. Treatment was conservative, through physiotherapy including passive and active shoulder exercises. The patient made an uneventful recovery, and 9 weeks after trauma he had full range of active and passive shoulder motions, with only minor discomfort in the extremes of abduction and elevation. A slight prominent lump remained visible in more than 90° abduction. Three months following the electric shock, the patient successfully returned to his normal professional activities (57).

Bilateral scapular fracture is a rare injury, as a result of high-energy trauma or muscle spasms associated with epileptiform seizure or electrical shock. It is most frequently recorded site was the scapular body, followed by the glenoid fossa. CT scan, including 3D CT reconstruction, is extremely important for diagnosis and assessment (45, 61, 63).

A 54-year-old man suffered accidentally a 240-voltage electric shock, through both hands as entry and exit points. He complained of awful upper back pain, without any direct trauma to his back. Initial assessments of respiratory, cardiovascular and neurologic functions were normal. Besides, he had partial thickness burns to his right hand with full range of movements and sensation. Inspection of his back was common, though it was very tender on palpation in the scapular, interscapular and infrascapular areas. Passive movements of both shoulder joints were extremely painful. Series X-rays of the cervical spine and the pelvis were normal. A portable chest radiograph showed probable scapular discontinuity on one side. The patient required pain medication and subsequent scapular radiographs and CT scan confirmed bilateral scapular fractures. He was referred to a tertiary centre for definitive management (73).

A 51-year-old engineer sustained a 240-voltage electric shock, through his left arm, across the shoulders and down the right arm, for 15-20 seconds, without fall or loss of consciousness. On emergency, he complained of severe pain in both shoulders. Nervous and cardiovascular examinations were normal, but he was very tender over the scapulae with restriction of shoulder movements bilaterally. X-rays revealed bilateral extra-articular fractures of the scapulae. EKG was normal, but blood tests showed elevated creatine kinase. He was admitted for cardiac monitoring and pain relief medication. A CT scan of his shoulders was performed to assess the extent of his fractures and to rule out any intra-articular extensions of the fractures. His bilateral scapular fractures were treated non-operatively in slings, with progressive physiotherapy and analgesia. He was discharged on day 10 and three months after the injury he was pain-free and had obtained a full range of movements in both shoulders (58).

Another 43-year-old man sustained bilateral scapular fractures following 440-voltage electrical exposure, passing briefly through his upper extremities, without fall or other direct trauma. The conservative treatment, consisting of shoulder immobilization, analgesia, and progressive physical therapy, led to healing of the fractures over six weeks, with restoration of the normal shoulder function after a follow-up period of six months (62).

Studies found in literature highlight indications for surgical treatment of scapular fracture, including glenoid fractures with dislocation or displacement of the fragments, and coracoid fracture with acromioclavicular separation or associated neuromuscular injury (59).

Maybe the most common osteoarticular injury detected after electrocution is **posterior fracture-dislocation of the shoulder** due to massive contraction of the infraspinatus and teres minor, with deltoid, latissimus dorsi and teres major forcing the humeral head superiorly and posteriorly against the acromion, and medially against the glenoid fossa, causing the humeral head to lodge behind the glenoid rim (56). It is important to keep in mind that this type of injury from electric shock can occur where there are no direct traumas and can be caused by violent muscular contractions. Once the patient is hemodynamically stabilised, the treatment of the osteoarticular injuries should follow the normal principles of orthopaedic surgery, aiming to achieve articular congruency through the reduction of the fragments, stable osteosyntheses and a normal functioning of the shoulder, and rehabilitation should begin at an early stage (74).

Thus, a 48-year-old man suffered a 500-voltage electrocution between both hands, without falling to the ground or experiencing loss of consciousness. On admission to the emergency department, the patient was conscious and oriented, in good general state and cardiopulmonary examination was normal. There were no burns on the body surface to be examined. He complained of severe pain and loss of function on the active mobilization of the right shoulder, presenting the arm abducted, with local swelling of the joint. The physical examination did not

43

evidence neurovascular deficits. The performed X-rays highlighted posterior dislocation of the humeral head. The first therapeutic attitude was to monitor the patient to rule out heart rhythm disorders, at the same time with the procedures for reducing orthopedic shoulder dislocation, which was immobilized with Dessault bandage. CT scan allowed to more accurately assess the glenohumeral joint, appreciating a broken head parcel remaining nestled in the back rim of the glenoid. Osteosynthesis was performed with cancellous screws, through shoulder anteromedial surgical approach (according to Thompson technique). Postoperative radiographs highlighted reducing of bony fragments, as well as correct joint congruence. One month after surgery, the rehabilitation service initiated passive and active shoulder mobilization. A year after the intervention, the patient had normal active life, returned to his work, although he had limited shoulder mobility in its last degrees of rotation (74).

Another 52-year-old man complained of pain and functional impotence of the right upper limb, due to electrical shock from a home device that was repaired, without fall or trauma to the affected limb. He was in good general condition and had no burns on the body. On emergency, physical examination revealed contraction of the scapulohumeral muscles and loss of function, but no motor or sensitive deficits. X-rays and CT scan of the right arm highlighted an **anterior scapulohumeral fracture-dislocation**. The patient was admitted and assessed for metabolic disorders and heart rate. At 12 hours after admission, closed reduction of shoulder dislocation was performed and hemiarthroplasty was scheduled, which consisted of placing Neer type prosthesis through a deltopectoral approach, with repairing of the tuberosity. The patient had a good postoperative evolution and he improved with a 20.8 DASH score and range of mobility of 100° anterior flexion, 90° abduction, 20° extension, 85° internal rotation and 10° external rotation, at 18 months after surgery (75).

The shoulder is the joint most frequently affected by dislocations, of which 98% are anterior, 2% are posterior and 1% is associated with fractures. Anterior dislocations and proximal humeral fractures (greater tuberosity and subcapital fractures) are readily diagnosed by clinical and complementary examinations. However, posterior shoulder dislocations are more difficult to diagnose, because the radiographic examination reveal only very subtle changes that can easily go unnoticed. As described in literature, posterior shoulder dislocations can pass undiagnosed up to months. Therefore, all patients suffering an electrical shock should be suspected and checked for posterior shoulder dislocation. The final outcome greatly depends on the timeliness of diagnosis, leading to prompt and adequate treatment. In a series of five posterior shoulder dislocations after electrocution, the authors performed McLaghlin technique in one case, with good result, and joint stabilization through pins in four cases, of which one attained an excellent result; two achieved a good result and other regular. Open surgery was used in only one patient (75, 76).

The most common mechanism of anterior shoulder dislocation is forced extension, abduction and external rotation. The greater tuberosity acts as a lever on the acromion, moving the humeral head out of glenoid cavity. In electrocutions, violent and uncoordinated contraction of the muscular groups of the scapula-humeral girdle can produce dislocation joint. When the discharge occurs on the upper limb in adduction and internal rotation, posterior dislocation is an effect of the internal rotators (latissimus dorsi, pectoralis major and subscapularis muscles). If the discharge occurs on the limb in flexion, abduction and external rotation, the anterior dislocation is an effect of the external rotators (infraspinatus and teres minor muscles). Therefore, the excessive muscular contractions in cases of electrocution, epilepsy, and electroconvulsive therapy lead more frequently to posterior shoulder dislocations, due to the relative strength of the internal rotators of shoulder compared to the external rotators. Moreover, a correct anamnesis and physical examination, as well as at least one shoulder anteroposterior and axillary X-ray are essential to evaluate the joint. Also, a CT scan provides a complete description of the lesion and may be very important to plan surgery (64, 75, 76).

The reduction of shoulder dislocation should be performed as soon as possible, to minimize the vascular lesion of the humeral head that can lead to osteonecrosis and subsequent colaps (60, 75). However, although perfusion of the head fragment is an essential element, it is not unique for the decision. Although in the presence of ischemic humeral head, conservative treatment is an option when revascularization is expected or when a management protocol of two stages is required: first stage osteosynthesis; second stage, hemiarthroplasty if avascular necrosis is not tolerated. In case of acute displaced fractures in young patients, gentle closed reduction is attempted; however, open reduction and internal fixation are the best option. If good result cannot be achieved or when more than 50% of the articular surface of the head is damaged, hemiarthroplasty is another therapeutic alternative. Some authors suggest that hemiarthroplasty is the treatment of choice in elderly patients (> 65 years) with comminuted fractures of the humeral head (three or four fragments), who are at high risk of avascular necrosis. However, others consider that there is insufficient evidence to establish that the hemiarthroplasty is a better therapeutic option than plate fixation (59, 75-79).

Bilateral posterior shoulder dislocation is a particular and rare situation, with different aetiologies, representing less than 5% of all posterior dislocations. The "triple E syndrome" (epilepsy or any convulsive seizure, extreme trauma and electric shock) represents the three most frequent causes of bilateral posterior shoulder dislocation. Almost 50% of bilateral posterior dislocations are due to a convulsive seizure, rising to 90% if the dislocations are associated with fractures, and less than 5% of them are caused by electric shocks. The diagnosis of bilateral posterior shoulder dislocation is often delayed, and up to

50% of them are not correctly identified on emergency. Accurate anamnesis, physical examination with at least one anteroposterior and one axillary X-rays are essential when assessing any shoulder complaint. Physical examination can ascertain normal contour of the shoulder, with a prominent coracoid process. Painful abnormal movement at the fracture site may be mistaken for normal glenohumeral movement. Possible associated nerve and vascular injuries should be verified. CT scan also provides a complete description of the lesion and can be valuable for planning surgery. Orthopaedic treatment should be performed according to the type of lesion, to the interval of time elapsed from the accident, and also to the age, occupation and desired levels of activity of the patient. Good results can be expected only if the anatomy is respected and if the procedure provides a stable joint. When the fracture is minimally displaced and the viability of the humeral head is not in doubt, closed reduction, and if necessary pin fixation, should be done, but at three weeks after trauma, closed reduction is almost impossible and surgical treatment is required. For displaced acute fractures in young patients, if an attempt of gentle closed reduction is not successful, open reduction and internal fixation is required. If open reduction cannot be achieved or in cases in which more than 50% of the joint surface of the humeral head is damaged, then hemiarthroplasty is recommended. In older patients (>65 years) with three or four-part acute fractures, there is a high risk of avascular necrosis, hence the indication is hemiarthroplasty. A total shoulder arthroplasty may be required, in case of both involvement of humeral head and glenoid damage (59, 64, 78-85).

Moreover, a Cochrane systematic review, published in 2015, showed that surgery does not result in a better outcome for the majority of patients with displaced proximal humeral fractures and is likely to result in a greater need for subsequent surgery. Otherwise, there is not enough evidence to determine the best non-surgical or, when selected, surgical treatment for these fractures (86).

Thus, a 56-year old man suffered a low-voltage electrical injury, with partial thickness burns at the level of his left hand, approximately 0.5% body surface, without fall or loss of consciousness. As usually, the burned wounds were debrided and sterile dressings with topical antiseptics were applied on the left hand. On admission, EKG, the pulmonary radiologic assessment and the usual blood tests were in normal range. The patient also complained of pain and functional impairment at the level of his left shoulder and proximal arm, which presented swelling, oedema and tenderness. The patient was unable to completely and actively elevate his left arm. Two days later, the shoulder X-ray highlighted comminuted subcapital fracture of the left humerus (Fig. 1). The orthopaedic surgeon recommended conservative treatment for humeral fracture, by closed reduction and immobilization through thoraco-brachial bandage for 30 days. The burned wounds evolution was good and the patient was discharged the fourth day, with subsequent complete epithelisation in other two weeks (87).

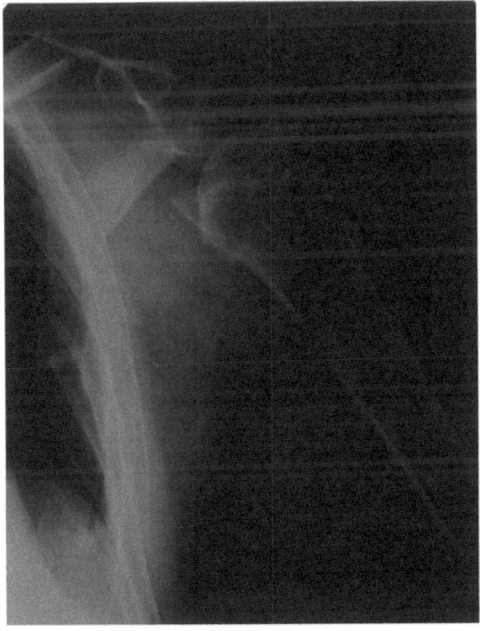

Figure 1. Comminuted subcapital fracture of the left humerus

Since bone has the highest electrical resistance among all body tissues, it also accumulates the greatest heat while conducting an electric current. This excessove heat can lead to osteonecrosis, an outstanding but less frequent complication of electric shock, most likely caused by bone "melting". Humeral head steonecrosis caused by electrical injury has been reported in the literature, in a case of a 52-year-old woman who had received 220-voltage electric shock (alternating household current) to the right hand and developed osteonecrosis in the ipsilateral humeral head. Therefore, an osteonecrotic lesion may develop in a distant joint towards the entry point, and this should always be remembered in the diagnosis and treatment of electrocuted patients (82, 88).

Most of fractures after electrically-induced tetanic muscle contractions involve the proximal appendicular skeleton, while distal fractures of limbs are uncommon. All forearm fractures reported in literature involved paediatric patients and suggest children vulnerability to this type of fracture (67), which could be attributed to factors such as:
-   initial electrical flow path through hand and forearm
-   more fragile paediatric bone structure

- less developed musculature of pectoral girdle in children, avoiding shoulder fractures as a result of strong muscle contractions.

Following low-voltage electric shocks, forearm fracture can occur at different levels, according to literature data:
- radius, in a 14-year-old boy who suffered also a minor burn (65)
- distal radius, unilateral in a 6 year-old girl (89) or bilateral, in a 12 year-old boy (14)
- wrist fracture, in a 6-year-old girl (89)
- Galeazzi fracture dislocation of the wrist (distal radius fracture with radioulnar joint disruption), in a 11-year old child (66)

Thus, a 6-year-old girl suffered local superficial burns of the right hand and a distal radius buckle-type fracture, following an accidental 230-V electric shock, without fall or loss of consciousness. The girl was touching with the right hand the metallic stand of a non-insulated street lamp, and then she felt a sudden jolt and managed to pull her hand free quickly. The superficial burns of the right hand were in accordance with electric marks, while the buckle fracture of the distal radius can be attributed to a sudden and powerful contraction of the flexor muscles of the hand (67).

Another 6-year-old girl suffered an accidental 230-volt electric shock, after touching also the stand of a non-insulated street lamp with her right hand. X-ray of the right wrist highlighted a distal fracture of the radius with an anterior displacement. The girl was conservatively treated and recovered normally after a three-week casting of the wrist articulation (89).

These paediatric cases are original due to the unusual localization of the fracture following low-voltage electrical shock. They emphasize the importance of careful and watchful physical examination and of complementary imaging studies in case of evident osteoarticular clinical symptoms and signs, after an electric shock at low-voltages, associated with falling or significant muscular contractures (89).

48

Chapter 10 Osteoarticular injuries of the pelvis and lower limb

Following electric shock, most osteoarticular injuries can be detected in the upper extremities, especially the shoulders. Further injuries include fractures of the vertebral bodies, scapular fractures, and femoral fractures (51). In patients without falling or loss of consciousness, the proximal femoral fractures can be related to violent muscle contractions of powerful pelvitrochanteric muscles, due to electrical current passage.

Thus, a 41-year old electrician suffered an accidental electrical shock with 300 V direct current, passing between his left hand and his left heel, without loss of consciousness. He then complained of pain at his left hip, and he was not able to stand or walk. He presented also two small full thickness burns under his left heel, probably the exit marks of the electrical current. At the emergency department, he was stable, EKG was normal and CK levels were slightly elevated. X-ray highlighted a **femoral neck fracture** on the left side, which was surgically treated the same day through open reduction and ostheosyntesis with a dynamic hip screw. The electric flow probably implicated only the left side of his body. After a year, the patient had completely recovered and a control X-ray evidenced no signs of malunion or avascular necrosis (51).

Simultaneous **bilateral femoral neck fractures** are extremely rare and have been associated with (52, 90):
- high energy trauma
- repetitive minor trauma
- abnormal anatomy
- irradiation for malignancy
- seizure
- electrical injury
- electroconvulsive therapy
- primary or secondary bone diseases: osteomalacia, hyperparathyroidism, chronic renal failure or severe osteoporosis, especially after corticotherapy.

According to literature data, the simultaneous bilateral hip fractures occur more commonly after electroconvulsive therapy rather than seizures, and with a male predominance. This could be explained by better development of the muscular structures surrounding the hip in the male. During convulsions, the powerful muscular contractions could lead to hip (including acetabular) fractures or dislocations (91).

Following electrical shock, bilateral femoral neck fractures are extremely rare and can appear even in the absence of primary and secondary bone disease (52-54, 92).

Thus, a 25-year-old man with no known previous medical disease was admitted two days after accidental electrical shock which occurred while he was trying to repair a 220 V air-conditioner, after initial treatment in a local hospital. X-ray films showed bilateral subcapital fracture of the femur, without other injuries or blood test abnormalities. Simultaneous bilateral open reduction and internal fixation were performed, using a nail and plate. The postoperative recovery was satisfactory and the patient was allowed to walk with a frame, at 3 weeks after the operation. He was discharged home after 6 weeks, and at 1 year had complete recovery and a full range of hip movement without symptoms. A follow-up X-ray film revealed good union (53).

Another 20-years old man accidentally suffered a 440 V direct current discharge, by putting his left hand on an electric wire with and getting stuck to it for several seconds. Thereafter, he fell backwards on his buttocks from standing height and he had a snapping sensation in both hips before falling, but did not lose consciousness. Then he complained of pain of both hips and could not stand or walk. At the emergency department, he was stable and had one small full-thickness burn on each heel, probably the exit wounds of the electrical flow. X-rays highlighted bilateral femoral neck fractures (Garden type 3). EKG and blood tests were normal. A complete history and general physical examination show no risk factors for any pathological fracture. Both femoral neck fractures were surgically treated within 24 hours of admission, through a limited approach and insertion of 3 cannulated screws into both femoral heads. He was mobilized postoperatively, allowed partial weight bearing and discharged after 12 days. He was allowed full weight bearing 3 weeks after surgery. The fractures healed with complete functional recovery in hips and no signs of malunion or avascular necrosis occur at 16 months' follow-up (52).

Different procedures have been reported in the literature for treatment of bilateral femoral neck fracture, single or in combination, such as (93, 94):
   - in situ fixation
   - open reduction and internal fixation, the most used option
   - open fixation with valgus intertrochanteric osteotomy
   - pedicle bone grafting
   - hemi or total hip arthroplasty in one or two-staged operations.
The postoperative complications include: non-union, delayed union and shortening. Femoral head osteonecrosis and coxa vara can be avoided with correct treatment (93).

The emergency physicians, orthopaedic surgeons and general practitioners should be particularly vigilant to the possibility of bilateral femoral neck fractures in electric injury patient, even in absence of high impact injury, primary or secondary bone disease, especially if the patients are confused and unable to standing, walk or localize pain. A delay in diagnosis is usual, and undiagnosed femoral neck fractures have deleterious long-term results and complications, which are common in young patient (52):

- pain
- risk of non-union and osteonecrosis of femoral head with functional disability
- degenerative joint disease
- progression of an undisplaced femoral neck fracture to a displaced fracture, due to a delayed diagnosis, which complicates the situation further.

A long-term systematic follow-up is recommended in all patients, with frequent clinical and X-ray check-ups, to evaluate their evolution and to avoid possible complications (52).

Early recognition and prompt surgical intervention of skeletal fractures following electrical injuries can lead to good outcomes. However, a delay in diagnosis is common, and a thorough and complete physical examination of the musculoskeletal system should therefore be performed in the patients with a high index of suspicion. X-ray studies are often unnecessary in alert cooperative patients with no significant tenderness, full active range of motion of the joints, and good function. In confuse, unconscious or uncooperative patients, X-ray studies of the shoulders, spine, and pelvis are indicated if these structures were in the path of the electric flow. Furthermore, in young patients, complications after femoral neck fractures are common and should be avoided by prompt diagnosis, suitable treatment and frequent postoperative checkups (51, 52).

In literature, electrical shock was also reported to determine the appearance of **osteonecrosis of the femoral head**, a disabling and devastating injury, which is not a specific entity, but the final common pathway of various conditions that impair the blood supply to the femoral head. Its pathogenesis is considered to be multifactorial and is associated in some cases with both, a genetic predilection and exposure to certain risk factors, such as:
- corticosteroid use
- alcohol intake
- smoking
- different chronic diseases: renal disease, hematological diseases, inflammatory bowel disease, hypertension and gout
- inherited coagulation disorders, thrombophilic and hypofibrinolytic coagulation abnormalities. These subclinical coagulation defects could result in a clinical disease when overlapped by environmental factors, the so called "second hit" (e.g., trauma, alcoholism, steroids) (95, 96).

In high voltage exposures, the electric current have a direct path between an entry and an exit point and induces severe injuries to blood vessels, nerves, muscles and skin, leading to soft tissues extensive damage and possible amputations at different levels. The radiological findings of these injuries which are thought to be pathognomonic include osteoschisis and bone pearls. Low voltage currents travel through the path of least resistance along nerves and blood vessels, since the bone is a poor conductor to electrical currents.

Osteonecrosis detected at a site distant to the entry or exit point is most likely attributed to injury to the vascular wall which in turn will cause thrombosis and ischemia. The effects of electrical injuries to bone may appear immediately or after a delay of months to years; in addition, the bony injuries may occur near the entry point or in the distance from contact points (95, 96).

Thus, a 39-years-old man suffered 220 volts electrocution to his left foot for less than one minute, without going to emergency department at that time. About two years later, he complained of hobbling and increasing chronic pain in the left hip and. He denied any history of trauma to the left hip and he has never taken steroids, smoked or consumed alcohol. A further detailed medical history did not reveal blood disorders or other diseases associated with osteonecrosis of the femoral head. Physical examination evidenced restricted and painful range of motion of the left hip. Blood tests were in normal range, including full blood count, liver function tests and coagulation screen, and serology for HIV, HBV, and HCV was negative. X-ray of the left hip highlighted advanced degenerative changes of the left hip joint with narrowing of the joint space, and a diagnosis of osteonecrosis of the femoral head was established. The patient was treated by total hip replacement, with good follow-up at five months. In this case, previous electrical discharge could damage the blood supply to the femoral head and lead to osteonecrosis of the femoral head. (95).

Another 36-years-old patient, which was carrier of a (heterozygous) prothrombin gene mutation, suffered 500 voltage electrocution to the right lower leg, which lead to osteonecrosis of the ipsilateral femoral head 18 months later. The authors suggest that an electrical exposure to his lower limb may have triggered intravascular thrombosis as a result of this mutation, with subsequent osteonecrosis of the femoral head (96).

Conclusions

Electrical aggressions are severe, destructive and disabling injuries, which are possibly fatal and can determine extensive skin and soft tissues damages, different organs and systems dysfunctions, various osteoarticular injuries and even amputations.

Electrical exposures can lead to unfrequently, but overlooked skeletal injuries, such as long bone fractures, spine fractures, joint dislocations, very deep burns, osteonecrosis and heterotopic ossification of soft tissues.

Since bone has the highest resistance of any body tissue, it also generates the greatest amount of heat when exposed to an electrical shock. Thereafter, the areas of greatest thermal damage are frequently the deep tissue surrounding long bones, resulting in periosteal burns, destruction of bone matrix, and osteonecrosis, besides extensive soft tissues injuries, which require aggressive medical therapy and serial surgical debridements. The resulting destruction is usually difficult to assess at the time of initial debridement. In such cases, stripping of the devitalized periosteum and obtaining early soft tissue coverage can limit the magnitude of bony injury (97).

Fractures and dislocations usually occur after a traumatic event related to electrical injuries, and they can be rarely caused by violent tetanic muscle contractions, as result of electrical current passage. Although fractures due to low-voltage electric discharge are rare, it should be borne in mind that after electric shock the presence of pain, swelling, bone tenderness, and impossibility or limitation of motion may be due to fractures. In all cases of electrical injury, the patients should be examined carefully and in detail (59).

Therefore, all practitioners involved in the management of the electrocuted patients need to be informed and to take account of the possibility of skeletal injuries: plastic surgeon, general surgeon, orthopaedic surgeon, emergency physician and general practitioner. To avoid a possible delay in diagnosis, the detailed and complete physical examination of the musculoskeletal system should be practiced in the electrocuted patients with suggestive symptoms and signs. The early recognition, the confirmation by X-ray examination and the prompt orthopaedic treatment ensure a favourable outcome and remove the harmful complications.

Treatment of fractures and dislocations should be indicated and performed in each particular case by the orthopaedic surgeon. The reduction of dislocation-fractures, adequate stabilization, and the restoration of normal functionality are the main objectives (81). For a good anatomic and functional outcome, as well as to avoid possible detrimental complications, the patients who underwent reconstructive skeletal surgery should be under close follow-up, and periodic clinical and radiologic assessments may be recommended (97).

References

1. WHO: Burns. Fact sheet N°365. Updated April 2014. Available from http://www.who.int/mediacentre/factsheets/fs365/en/. Accessed at 20.12.2015.

2. WHO: Violence and Injury Prevention. Burns. Available from http://www.who.int/violence_injury_prevention/other_injury/burns/en/. Accessed at 20.12.2015.

3. American Burn Association: Burn Incidence and Treatment in the United States: 2015. Available from http://www.ameriburn.org/resources_factsheet.php. Accessed at 20.12.2015

4. American Burn Association: Burn Center Referral Criteria. Available from http://www.ameriburn.org/BurnCenterReferralCriteria.pdf. Accessed at 20.12.2015

5. Carter JE, Neff LP, Holmes JH. Adherence to burn center referral criteria: are patients appropriately being referred? J Burn Care Res. 2010; 31(1):26-30

6. British Burn Association Standards. European Standards. Available from http://www.britishburnassociation.org/european-standards. Accessed at 20.12.2015

7. Cushing TA, Wright RK. Electrical Injuries in Emergency Medicine. Available from http://emedicine.medscape.com/article/770179-overview. Updated: Jul 31, 2015. Accessed at 20.12.2015

8. Lee RC, Zhang D, Hannig J. Biophysical injury mechanisms in electrical shock trauma. Annu Rev Biomed Eng. 2000; 02:477–509.

9. Daley BJ, Mallat AF, Goycolea JFA, Gallegos JJ. Electrical Injuries. Available from http://emedicine.medscape.com/article/433682-overview. Updated: May 09, 2014. Accessed at 20.12.2015

10. Purdue GF, Arnoldo BD, Hunt JL. Chapter 39. Electrical injuries. p. 513-520. In Herndon DN, editor. Total Burn Care. IIIrd edition. Philadelphia: Saunders Elsevier, 2007.

11. Vogt PM, Niederbichler AD, Spies M, Muehlberger T. Chapter 40. Electrical injury: reconstructive problems. p. 521-529. In Herndon DN, editor. Total Burn Care. IIIrd edition. Philadelphia: Saunders Elsevier, 2007.

12. Young DM. Chapter 29. Burn and electrical injury. In: Mathes S, editor. Plastic Surgery. Philadelphia: Saunders Elsevier, 2006. p. 831

13. Dzhokic G, Jovchevska J, Dika A. Electrical injuries: etiology, pathophysiology and mechanism of injury. Maced J Med Sci. 2008; 1(2):54-58.

14. Stone N, Karamitopoulos M, Edelstein D, Hashem J, Tucci J. Bilateral distal radius fractures in a 12-year-old boy after household electrical shock: case report and literature summary. Case Rep Med. 2014; 2014: 235756.

15.   Ungureanu M. Electrocutions – treatment strategy (case presentation). J Med Life. 2014; 7(4): 623–626.

16.   Hussmann J, Kucan JO, Russell RC, Bradley T, Zamboni WA. Electrical injuries - morbidity, outcome and treatment rationale. *Burns.* 1995; 21(7): 530-5355.

17.   Jensen PJ, Thomsen PE, Bagger JP, Nørgaard A, Baandrup U. Electrical injury causing ventricular arrhythmias. *Br Heart J.* 1987; 57(3): 279-283.

18.   Claudet I, Marechal C, Debuisson C, Salanne S. Risque de trouble du rythme et électrisation par courant domestique [Risk of arrhythmia and domestic low-voltage electrical injury]. *Arch Pediatr.* 2010; 17(4): 343-349.

19.   Yang JY, Tsai YC, Noordhoff MS. Electrical burn with visceral injury. Burns Incl Therm Inj. 1985; 11(3): 207–212.

20.   Branday JM, DuQuesnay DR, Yeesing MT, Duncan ND. Visceral complications of electrical burn injury. A report of two cases and review of the literature. West Indian Med J. 1989; 38(2):110–113.

21.   Honda T, Yamamoto Y, Mizuno M, Mitsusada M, Nakazawa H, Sasaki K, Nozaki M. Successful treatment of a case of electrical burn with visceral injury and full-thickness loss of the abdominal wall. Burns. 2000; 26(6):587-592.

22.   Bailey B, Gaudreault P, Thivierge RL. Cardiac monitoring of high-risk patients after an electrical injury: a prospective multicentre study. *Emerg Med J.* 2007; 24(5):348-352.

23.   Dollery W. Towards evidence based emergency medicine: best BETs from the Manchester Royal infirmary. Management of household electrical injury. *J Accid Emerg Med.* 1998; 15(4):228.

24.   Chen EH, Sareen A. Do children require ECG evaluation and inpatient telemetry after household electrical exposures? *Ann Emerg Med.* 2007; 49(1):64-67.

25.   Kopp J, Loos B, Spilker G, Horch RE. Correlation between serum creatinine kinase levels and extent of muscle damage in electrical burns. *Burns.* 2004; 30(7):680-683.

26.   Rosen CL, Adler JN, Rabban JT, Sethi RK, Arkoff L, Blair JA, Sheridan R. Early predictors of myoglobinuria and acute renal failure following electrical injury. *J Emerg Med.* 1999; 17(5):783-789.

27.   Teodoreanu R, Popescu S, Lascar I. Electrical injuries. Biological values measurements as a prediction factor of local evolution in electrocutions lesions. Journal of Medicine and Life. 2014; 7(2): 226-236.

28.   Arnoldo B, Klein M, Gibran NS. Practice guidelines for the management of electrical injuries. *J Burn Care Res.* 2006; 27(4):439-447.

29.   Warden GD. Chapter 9. Fluid resuscitation and early management. p. 197-118. In Herndon DN, editor. Total Burn Care. IIIrd edition. Philadelphia: Saunders Elsevier, 2007.

30. Mann R, Gibran N, Engrav L, Heimbach D. Is immediate decompression of high voltage electrical injuries to the upper extremity always necessary? J Trauma. 1996; 40(4):584–587.

31. Yowler CJ, Mozingo DW, Ryan JB, Pruitt BA. Factors contributing to delayed extremity amputation in burn patients. J Trauma. 1998; 45(3):522–526.

32. Bartle EJ, Wang XW, Miller GJ. Early vascular grafting to prevent upper extremity necrosis after electrical burns: anastomotic false aneurysm, a severe complication. Burns Incl Therm Inj. 1987; 13(4):313–317.

33. Wang XW, Bartle EJ, Roberts BB, Cheng HH, Wu WA, Wang XZ. Free skin flap transfer in repairing deep electrical burns. J Burn Care Rehabil 1987; 8(2):111–4.

34. Johnson EV, Klein LB, Skalka HW. Electrical cataracts: a case report and review of the literature. Ophthalmic Surg. 1987; 18:283–285.

35. Boozalis GT, Purdue GF, Hunt JL, McCulley JP. Ocular changes from electrical burn injuries: a literature review and report of cases. J Burn Care Rehabil. 1991; 5:458–462.

36. Mutlu FM, Duman H, Cli Y. Early-onset unilateral electric cataract: a rare clinical entity. J Burn Care Rehabil 2004; 25:363–365.

37. Saffle JR, Crandall A, Warden GD. Cataracts: a long-term complication of electrical injury. J Trauma. 1985; 25:17.

38. Grube BJ, Heimbach DM, Engrav LH, Copass MK. Neurologic consequences of electrical burns. J Trauma. 1990; 30:254–258.

39. Haberal MA, Gürer S, Akman N, Başgöze O. Persistent peripheral nerve pathologies in patients with electric burns. J Burn Care Rehabil. 1996; 17:147–149.

40. Barrasch J. Neurologic and neurobehavioral effects of electric and lightning injuries. J Burn Care Rehabil. 1996; 17:409.

41. Janus TJ, Barrash J. Neurologic and neurobehavioural effects of electric and lightning injuries. J Burn Care Rehabil. 1996; 17:409–415.

42. Pliskin NH, Capelli-Schellpfeffer M, Law RT, Malina AC, Kelley KM, Lee RC. Neuropsychological symptom presentation after electrical injury. J Trauma. 1998; 44:709–715.

43. Luz DP, Millan LS, Alessi MS, Uguetto WF, Paggiaro A, Gomez DS, Ferreira MC. Electrical burns: a retrospective analysis across a 5-year period. *Burns*. 2009: 35(7):1015-1019.

44. Bracken TD, Kavet R, Patterson RM, Fordyce TA. An integrated job exposure matrix for electrical exposures of utility workers. *J Occup Environ Hyg*. 2009; 6(8):499-509.

45. Dumas JL, Walker N. Bilateral scapular fractures secondary to electrical shock. Arch Orthop Trauma Surg. 1992; 111:287–288.

46. Adams AJ, Beckett MW. Bilateral wrist fractures from accidental electric shock. Injury. 1997; 28:227–228.

47.   Tompkins GS, Henderson RC, Peterson HD. Bilateral simultaneous fractures of the femoral neck: case report. J Trauma. 1990; 30:1415–1416.

48.   Van den Brink WA, van Leeuwen O. Lumbar burst fracture due to low voltage shock. A case report. Acta Orthop Scand. 1995; 66:374–375.

49.   Helm PA, Walker SC. New bone formation at amputation in electrically burn-injured patients. Arch Phys Med Rehabil. 1987; 68:284–286.

50.   Alexander WN. Composite dysplasia of a single tooth as a result of electrical burn damage: report of a case. J Am Dent Assoc. 1961; 69:589.

51.   Gehlen JLMG, Hoofwijk AGM. Femoral neck fracture after electrical shock injury. Eur J Trauma Emerg Surg. 2010; 36(5): 491-493.

52.   Sohal HS, Goyal D. Simultaneous bilateral femoral neck fractures after electrical shock injury: a case report. Chin J Traumatol. 2013; 16(2):126-128.

53.   Shaheen MA, Sabet NA. Bilateral simultaneous fracture of the femoral neck following electrical shock. Injury. 1984; 16(1):13-14.

54.   Nabours RE, Fish RM, Hill PF. Electrical Injuries: Engineering, Medical and Legal Aspects. Second Edition. Lawyers & Judges Publishing Company, USA, 2004

55.   Slater RR, Peterson HD. Bilateral femoral neck fractures after electrical injury: a case report and literature review. J Burn Care Rehabil. 1990; 11(3):240-243.

56.   Rana M, Banerjee R. Scapular fracture after electric shock. Ann R Coll Surg Engl. 2006; 88(2): W3–W4.

57.   Simon JP, van Delm I, Fabry G. Comminuted fracture of the scapula following electric shock. A case report. Acta Orthopaedica Belgica. 1991; 57(4):459-460.

58.   Kotak BP, Haddo O, Iqbal M, Chissell H. Bilateral scapular fractures after electrocution. J R Soc Med. 2000; 93:143-144.

59.   Duman H, Kopal C, Selmanpakoglu N. Bilateral shoulder fracture following low-voltage electrical injury. Ann Burn Fire Dis. 2000; 13(3): 173-174.

60.   Tan AH. Missed posterior fracture-dislocation of the humeral head following an electrocution injury to the arm. Singapore Med J. 2005; 46(4):189-192.

61.   Tarquinio T, Weinstein ME, Virgilio RW. Bilateral scapular fractures from accidental electric shock. J Trauma. 1979; 19(2):132-133.

62.   Beswick DR, Morse SD, Barnes AU. Bilateral scapular fractures from low-voltage electrical injury. Ann Emerg Med. 1982; 11(12):676-677.

63.   Tuček M, Bartoníček J, Novotný P, Voldřich M. Bilateral scapular fractures in adults. Int Orthop. 2013; 37(4):659-665.

64.   Bachhal V, Goni V, Taneja A, Shashidhar BK, Bali K. Bilateral four-part anterior fracture dislocation of the shoulder - a case report and review of literature. Bull NYU Hosp Jt Dis. 2012; 70(4):268-272.

65.   Pappano D. Radius fracture from an electrical injury involving an electric guitar. South Med J. 2010; 103(3):242-244.

66.   Hostetler MA, Davis CO. Galeazzi fracture resulting from electrical shock. Pediatr Emerg Care. 2000; 16(4):258-259.

67.   Peyron PA, Cathala P, Vannucci C, Baccino E. Wrist fracture in a 6-year-old girl after an accidental electric shock at low voltages. Int J Legal Med. 2015; 129(2):297-300.

68.   Meschan I, Scruggs JB, Calhoun JD. Convulsive fractures of the dorsal spine following electric-shock therapy. Radiology. 1950; 54(2):180-193.

69.   Layton TR, McMurtry JM, McClain EJ, Kraus DR, Reimer BL. Multiple spine fractures from electric injury. J Burn Care Rehabil. 1984; 5:373-375.

70.   Sinha A, Dolakia M. Thoracic compression fracture caused by electrically induced injury. Physical Medicine and Rehabilitation. 2009; 1(8):780-782.

71.   Dolakia M, Sinha A. Spinal compression fracture caused by electrocution: A case report. Arch Phys Med Rehabil. 2008; 89:E72

72.   Hafidi J, El Mazouz S, El Mejatti H, Fejjal N, Gharib NE, Abbassi A, Belmahi AM. Lambeaux autofermants pour le traitement des brulures electriques du scalp par haut voltage. Ann Burns Fire Disasters. 2011; 24(2):72-76.

73.   John BS, Poyner F, Holloway V. Bilateral scapular fractures following low voltage electrocution. Grand Rounds. 2004; Vol 4: 10–12

74.   Esteo Pérez I, García Salama F, Zurita Uroz N, López Ortiz R, Valverde Cámara F. Fractura-luxación posterior de la cabeza humeral por electrocución [Posterior fracture-dislocation of the humeral head by electrocution]. Rev S And Traum Ort. 2001; 21(2):238-243.

75.   Ignacio Arzac Ulla, Edmundo Faiman, Marco Bolaños, Gonzalo Pérez Pa. Fractura de húmero proximal por descarga eléctrica - Reporte de un caso. Rev Asoc Argent Ortop Traumatol. 2014; 79(3): 190-192.

76.   Herrero Barcos L, Martínez Martín AA, Herrera Rodríguez A, Cuenca Espiérrez J, Panisello Sebastià JJ. Lesiones en el hombro causadas por electrocución. Revista Española de Cirugía Osteoarticular. 2001; 36:51-55.

77.   Breederveld RS, Patka P, Dwars BJ, Van Mourik JC. Shoulder injury caused by electric shock. Neth J Surg. 1987; 39(5):147-8.

78.   Cooke SJ, Hackney RG. Bilateral posterior four-part fracture-dislocations of the shoulders following electric shock: A case report and literature review. Injury. 2005; 36:90-95.

79.   Tey IK, Tan AHC. Posterior fracture-dislocation of the humeral head treated without the use of metallic implants. Singapore Med J. 2007; 48(4):e114-118.

80.   Claro R, Sousa R, Massada M, Ramos J, Lourenco J. Bilateral posterior fracture-dislocation of the shoulder: Report of two cases. Int J Shoulder Surg. 2009; 3(2):41-45.

81.   Sorando E, Agullo D, Garcia J, Amrouni B. Bilateral shoulder fractures secondary to accidental electrical injury. Case report. Ann Burns Fire Disasters. 2006; 19(1):41-43.

82.   Zumrut M, Marcil E. Bilateral shoulder injury caused by electric shock. JAEMCR. 2013; 4:92-94.

83.   Dinopoulos HT, Giannoudis PV, Smith RM, Matthews SJ. Bilateral anterior shoulder fracture-dislocation. A case report and review of the literature. Int Orthop. 1999; 23(2):128-130.

84.   Martens C, Hessels G. Bilateral posterior four-part fracture-dislocation of the shoulder. Acta Orthop Belg. 1995; 61:249-254.

85.   Clough T.M., Bale R.S. Bilateral posterior shoulder dislocation: The importance of the axillary radiographic view. Eur J Emerg Med. 2001; 8:161–163.

86.   Handoll HHG, Brorson S. Interventions for treating proximal humeral fractures in adults. *Cochrane Database of Systematic Reviews* 2015, Issue 11. Art. No.: CD000434.

87.   Zbuchea A. Humeral neck fracture after electrocution – case report and literature review. Chirurgia (Bucur). 2015; 110(5):490-492.

88.   Govoni M, Orzincolo C, Bigoni M, Feggi L, Pareschi PL, Trotta F. Humeral head osteonecrosis caused by electrical injury: a case report. J Emerg Med. 1993; 11(1):17-21.

89.   Peyron PA, Cathala P, Baccino E. Fractures osseuses par électrisations à basse tension: à propos de deux cas. La Revue de Medecine Legale. 2014; 5(4):170-175.

90.   Hootkani A, Moradi A, Vahedi E. Neglected simultaneous bilateral femoral neck fractures secondary to narcotic drug abuse treated by bilateral one-staged hemiarthroplasty: a case report. J Orthop Surg Res. 2010; 5: 41.

91.   Haronian E, Silver JW, Mesa J. Simultaneous bilateral femoral neck fracture and greater tuberosity shoulder fracture resulting from seizure. Orthopedics. 2002; 25(7):757-758.

92.   Nyoni L, Saunders CR, Morar AB. Bilateral fracture of the femoral neck as a direct result of electrocution shock. Cent Afr J Med. 1994; 40(12): 355-356.

93.   Hootkani A, Moradi A, Vahedi E. Neglected simultaneous bilateral femoral neck fractures secondary to narcotic drug abuse treated by bilateral one-staged hemiarthroplasty: a case report. J Orthop Surg Res. 2010; 5: 41.

94.   Grimaldi M, Vouaillat H, Tonetti J, Merloz P. Simultaneous bilateral femoral neck fractures secondary to epileptic seizures: Treatment by bilateral total hip arthroplasty. *Orthopaedics & Traumatology: Surgery & Research.* 2009; 95(7): 555-557.

95.   Abduljabbar FA, Mohammed J. Al-Sayyad MJ. Osteonecrosis of the femoral head triggered by an electrical injury. JKAU: Med. Sci. 2009; 16(3): 93-98,

96.   Vanderstraeten L, Binns M. Osteonecrosis of the femoral head following an electrical injury to the leg. J Bone Joint Surg Br. 2008; 90(8): 1101-1104.

97.   Imani MT, Mohammadi AA, Jafari SMS. Spontaneous fracture of the humerus 18 months after a high voltage electrical injury: A case report. Oman Med J. 2014; 29(2).

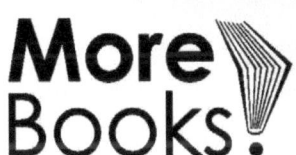

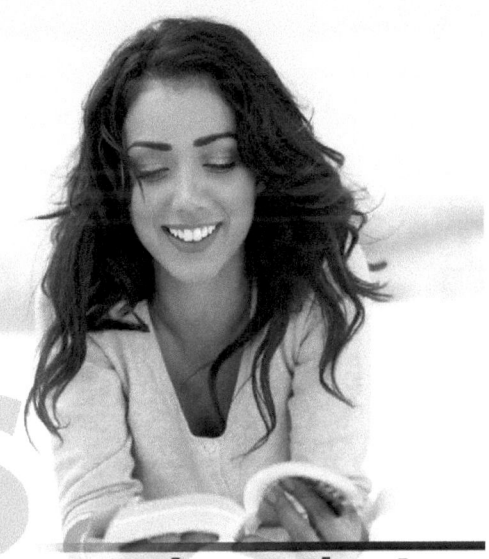

I **want** morebooks!

Buy your books fast and straightforward online - at one of the world's fastest growing online book stores! Environmentally sound due to Print-on-Demand technologies.

Buy your books online at
www.get-morebooks.com

Kaufen Sie Ihre Bücher schnell und unkompliziert online – auf einer der am schnellsten wachsenden Buchhandelsplattformen weltweit!
Dank Print-On-Demand umwelt- und ressourcenschonend produziert.

Bücher schneller online kaufen
www.morebooks.de

OmniScriptum Marketing DEU GmbH
Heinrich-Böcking-Str. 6-8
D - 66121 Saarbrücken
Telefax: +49 681 93 81 567-9

info@omniscriptum.com
www.omniscriptum.com

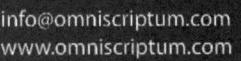
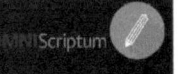

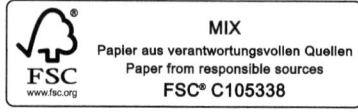

MIX
Papier aus verantwortungsvollen Quellen
Paper from responsible sources
FSC® C105338

Printed by Books on Demand GmbH, Norderstedt / Germany